Alex,

Thanks for your
early support and
for helping to save
the world.

The Karma Sense Eating Plan

Be Happy, Be Healthy, Save the World

David Hellman

 Karma Sense Eating Plan ™

Printed in the United States of America

First Printing, 2016

ISBN: 978-0-9971879-0-8 (collector's color paperback)
        978-0-9971879-1-5 (paperback)
        978-0-9971879-2-2 (ePub)
        978-0-9971879-3-9 (mobi)
        978-0-9971879-4-6 (PDF)

LiveLongLeadLong, LLC
407 E Nelson Ave
Alexandria, VA 22301

Although the author and publisher have made every effort to ensure that the information in this book was correct at press time, the author and publisher do not assume and hereby disclaim any liability to any party for any loss, damage, or disruption caused by errors or omissions, whether such errors or omissions result from negligence, accident, or any other cause.

The material in this book is for informational purposes only. As each individual situation is unique, you should use proper discretion, in consultation with a health care practitioner, before undertaking the nutrition and activity techniques described in this book. The author and publisher expressly disclaim responsibility for any adverse effects that may result from the use of application of the information contained in this book.

Links or references to external or third-party web sites are provided to readers solely as a convenience and are for informational purposes only; they do not constitute an endorsement or an approval by the author or publisher. The author and publisher bear no responsibility for the accuracy, legality, or content of the external site of for that of subsequent links. Contact the external site for answers to questions regarding its content.

Cover design by Richard Demler.

Edited by Jeanie Simoncic.

Author photograph by David Hellman.

Karma Sense® is a registered trademark of LiveLongLeadLong, LLC.

This book is dedicated to Susan Hellman, my driving instructor and love of my life,
to my debate coaches Sam and Travis Hellman, the products and targets of our love,
to Sheila and Abe Hellman, my teachers on how to love,
to every other teacher who ever taught me something even if it wasn't about love,
and to those crazy kids from Cohort 23.

All profits from the sale of this book are donated to charities that fight poverty and hunger. Learn more about our progress at
http://www.livelongleadlong.com/karma-sense/board/

Table of Contents

Prelims

Executive Summary (Introduction)

It may seem odd to begin an accessible manual for improving health and happiness with a chapter called *Executive Summary*. It's also strange for a high tech business executive and entrepreneur to write a book of this type and on this subject. But I'm a high tech business executive who also runs an Integrative Health Coaching practice targeted towards busy people. I'm certified by Precision Nutrition (PN) as an Exercise Nutrition coach (PN is one of the top ten most innovative companies in fitness[1]) and trained by Duke University Medical Center as an Integrative Health Coach (Duke is one of the top ten medical schools in the US.[2])

So I'm beginning this book the same way I begin most of what I write regardless of whether it's about technology or health; with a summary for busy people who want me to cut to the chase.

But an introductory executive summary is the only similarity between this book and stodgy business writing.

That's because this isn't a book about business. It's a book about you. It's a book that reacquaints you with how amazing food is. Reading this book will remind you that food is not only a source of nutrition but also a source of well-being. It's the source of your *entire* being. We were designed to enjoy food. Why else would our senses of smell and taste take up more DNA in our genetic code than any other body system?[3] Why else does the experience of tasting food light up more areas of the brain than any other behavior?[4] It's no wonder we collectively spend trillions of dollars each year to become healthier and happier, with much of that spending centered on food.[5]

When it comes to those trillions, many organizations would like to grab it from you. The biggest culprit is a loosely-knit faction comprised of corporations, "not-for-profit" institutions, and government entities that I call the Healthcare Industrial Complex (HIC). They're not all healthcare companies in the traditional sense, but they absolutely influence our health and often use health claims to sell their wares.

There's another group that sees right through the selfish motivation of the HIC. They understand that the HIC couldn't care less about your health or happiness. I call this other team the Healthy Lifestyle Militia (The Militia). The Militia knows that the HIC's true incentive is to keep you unhealthy and unhappy so that you continue to hand them more money. Unfortunately, many in The Militia are also motivated by self-interest. They're after their slice of the multi-trillion dollar pie and, their strategy is to take extreme and militant positions that simultaneously create false hope and FUD (fear, uncertainty, and doubt) to sell their products. These are the nutrition, exercise, and alternative health gurus who blanket all means of communication with wild claims that are either half-truths or totally unsubstantiated.

I represent neither of these factions. I'm not a doctor. I'm not a life scientist. I'm not a food industry insider. And I'm definitely not a celebrity health expert. I'm one of you. I'm a working stiff with a normal family living on Main Street, USA. I'm Ward Cleaver. I'm Mike Brady. I'm Tim Taylor, Danny Tanner, and Phil Dunphy.

I am all of these people. If they had an unnatural, irrational, and insatiable curiosity about physical health, mental health, and physiology, we'd be exactly the same. I am to those subjects as Richard Dreyfuss is to Devil's Tower in the movie *Close Encounters of the Third Kind*.

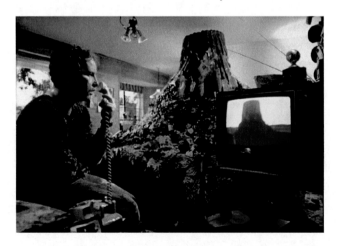

Figure 1 Richard Dreyfus obsessed with Devil's Tower[6,7]

I am totally obsessed.

Which leads me to one of my quirks; I have a way of tying obscure pop-culture references into just about every conversation. For example, I don't know why, to this day, I remember that Carl Douglas sang the 1975 hit "Kung Fu Fighting," yet I do.[8] It's just my superpower. Some of my references even manage to be current. Many may be more geared towards an eight-year-old than to you. You'll notice this as you read along.

But I don't want to minimize what I bring to the table. My training comes from two of the leading and most prestigious institutions in their respective fields. I've taken thousands of hours of courses on food, cooking, and the food business. I have magazines, books, and an e-mail inbox flooded with data on the subject—and I read them all. And when I'm not working my 6:00 am to 6:00 pm job in high technology, I practice as a health coach guiding athletes, business people, and other folks with hectic lives toward professional and personal success.

One night, after a long day of filling my roles as business executive and health coach, a revelation startled me awake. I realized that everything the HIC says is right. I also realized that everything The Militia says is right. They're also both very wrong. Each cherry-picks the data to make its case while ignoring the facts that allow us to call their claims bullcrap. But the truth is, the basic laws of chemistry, biology, physics, and math never change. And because of this, you only need to know a small and finite set of things to become the healthiest, happiest version of you.

This book, *The Karma Sense Eating Plan*, shares these basic truths. It allows you to assemble a plan for optimal health that conforms to your values, lifestyle, and schedule. Regardless of whether your diet preference is vegan, vegetarian, reducetarian (people who eat some meat; just not a lot of it), omnivore, or Paleo, you can apply *The Karma Sense Eating Plan* to improve your health.

Gluten-free? Yup! Dairy-free? Yes! Like your gluten and your dairy? Fer shizzle (which is how I believe the cool kids say "for sure," if they were saying it in the 1990s)! *The Karma Sense Eating Plan* does not require that you shop organic, avoid genetically modified organisms (GMOs), or eat only all-natural (whatever that means). There may be good reasons to eat this way. And that's up to you.

Furthermore, regardless of your religion or political affiliation, following the plan will make you happier. And it does so without depending on hopes, dreams, and guesses but instead uses what we know from hundreds of years of science. There's nothing wrong with hopes, dreams, and guesses if they do indeed make you happy. But it's nice to know that research backs up this stuff.

Oh yeah, let's not forget that *The Karma Sense Eating Plan* not only makes you healthier and happier but also gives you an opportunity to save the world. How's that for a side benefit?

The pages that follow describe the plan in detail. *The Karma Sense Eating Plan* is a sincere effort to improve your health, happiness, and as a byproduct, save the world. It's sincere, but it doesn't take itself too seriously. It demands nothing of you. It's a dogma-free, open source program for better health that you can adopt and adapt at your pleasure.

And know this: if you purchased this book and have read this far, you've already made progress in increasing your happiness and saving the world. According to one study,[9] purchasing experiential products such as books has a positive effect on your well-being. And as far as saving the world is concerned, I donate **all profits** from the sale of this book to charities that fight poverty and hunger (see In Closing… chapter at the end of the Appendix for more information on charitable donations).

I hope you enjoy your journey to becoming a happier and healthier version of you. I welcome your feedback and questions. And I apologize if you spend the rest of your day with a "Kung Fu Fighting" earworm.

Navigating *The Karma Sense Eating Plan*

Components

The Karma Sense Eating Plan consists of building blocks that are called *Components*. There are four components in total, and each gets its own section in the book. Each section consists of one or more chapters. The chapters can be read in any sequence, but I recommend that you do a quick scan of all the chapters and then decide which ones interest you. To simplify navigation, I include the following logos. They'll help you find the parts most relevant to you.

The components are called Karma, Sense, Eating, and Plan. When speaking about the entire plan together, you'll see this symbol:

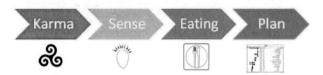

When focused on the Karma component, you'll see this:

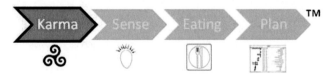

For the Sense component:

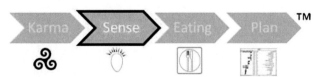

Eating component:

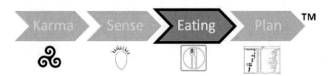

And Plan component:

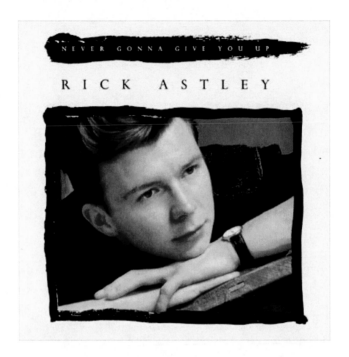

Figure 2 You've Been <u>Rickrolled</u>[10,11]

Ooops, sorry, I mean Plan component:

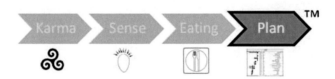

Higher Purpose

I created *The Karma Sense Eating Plan* because I want you to be healthier and happier. I also want to help save the world, but I can't do that without you. Somehow the remembering useless stuff superpower doesn't have a big effect in the world saving department ("Tell me who pitched when Roger Maris hit his record breaking home run or I'll destroy the world!").*

---

* Tracy Stallard

You may not believe that *The Karma Sense Eating Plan* can achieve all of these goals. I don't blame you. That's a tall order. Whenever I am trying to convince you that a particular chapter is focused on any of these three purposes, I'll use these symbols:

Symbol	How Does This Section Meet KSEP's Higher Purpose?		
	Healthy	Happy	Save the World
Healthy / Happy / Save the World	✓	✓	✓
Healthy / Happy / Save the World	✓		
Healthy / Happy / Save the World		✓	
Healthy / Happy / Save the World			✓
Healthy / Happy / Save the World	✓	✓	
Healthy / Happy / Save the World	✓		✓
Healthy / Happy / Save the World		✓	✓

Chapter Content

When appropriate, many chapters include the subsections described below to help you figure out if you should read the chapter in depth, skim it, or skip it. The subsection titles also serve as handy reminders if you read through the chapter once and want to touch on the salient points again.

Executive Summary

The Executive Summary is a narrative description of what is covered in the chapter.

Special Considerations

The Karma Sense Eating Plan may need some adjustments depending on what you are trying to achieve. When appropriate, Special Considerations covers these adjustments for some of the most common goals people have when they are trying to be healthier.

Key Points

The Key Points are bullet point summaries of what you need to do to honor the recommendations in the chapter.

Karma Sense in the Wild

Karma Sense in the Wild includes short stories about people's experiences implementing individual parts of *The Karma Sense Eating Plan*. These are real stories about real people although some people asked that I change identifying information because they're shy and they enjoy their privacy. For mantra #4, I end up with a composite of two characters but the results are real.

More Information

I continuously post updated information about *The Karma Sense Eating Plan* on my website. The site includes the original raw, unedited version of *The Karma Sense Eating Plan*. It also includes supplementary material often generated from user questions. You can find an index of all things Karma Sense at www.karma-sense.com.

Special Note for Print Version

One of the best features of *The Karma Sense Eating Plan* is its evidence-based approach to being happier, healthier, and saving the world. The plan depends heavily on research to support its claims. The electronic version of this book includes hyperlinks directly to the referenced studies. Unfortunately, we're still waiting for affordable electronic paper technology so those hyperlinks won't work in the print version.

If you want to review any of the studies or videos I reference in print, navigate to the notes at the end of the book and you'll find sufficient information to access these resources through an internet search.

Personally, I find the inability to click through directly from the print version an advantage. This way I can focus on what I'm reading without getting distracted by the latest cat video.

The *Karma Sense Eating Plan* Origin Story

Executive Summary

In the world of comic book superheroes, which is a passion of mine (shocker!), the *origin story* provides the critical background needed to appreciate the strengths and vulnerabilities of the characters.

This chapter is the origin story for *The Karma Sense Eating Plan* and the person inflicting it upon you. Reading this will help you decide how to interpret the rest of the book. Upon reading this chapter, some people will recognize that the plan distills the tidal wave of confusing and overly technical data that's supposed to improve your life, and presents it in an accessible and mildly amusing way. Others may decide I have no business writing a book on this or any other subject. Those in the latter group have the opportunity to laugh at me instead of laughing with me.

If you're not interested in the background and just want to jump into the heart of the matter, skip this chapter and move onto *The Karma Sense Eating Plan* Overview.

Either way, I encourage you to read the entire book. According to a Western Kentucky University study, laughter decreases stress and increases immune function.[12] And in a different study, even people who experienced catastrophic loss improve their happiness through laughter.[13] Here again, simply by reading *The Karma Sense Eating Plan*, your health and happiness will improve. Thus, even if you find it hard to take me seriously, you'll discover that I'm delivering on my promise of better health and happiness.

My Origin Story

My name is Dave Hellman. You'll learn more about me as you work your way through this book. I'm a late-stage baby boomer born in Brooklyn, New York, raised in suburban New Jersey, who spent adulthood in Durham, North Carolina; Los Angeles, California; and Northern Virginia. Because *David* was a common boy's name for my generation, many people call me *Davey H* to distinguish me from all the other Davids who were hanging around.

The following table presents some relevant personality quirks that I've had all my life and that the people who love me have come to accept.

Quirk	How It Manifests Itself in Life	How It Manifests Itself in This Book
Tendency towards being a wisenheimer	The first thing that comes out of my mouth is rarely serious.	This book is riddled with riddles, jokes, and random pop-culture references.
I am mildly on the Asperger's spectrum	I struggle to make judgments in the absence of fact. I've never been good at jumping to conclusions or trusting my "gut."	I don't like to make claims in this book unless I can back them up with facts and research. Some of the book's more amorphous subjects (e.g., karma) make this difficult.
	I try to systemize everything	You'll see a lot of tables and graphs in this book when narrative descriptions would do. Consider this table a case in point.
I am very empathetic	While people with Asperger's struggle with sympathy, we're much better with empathy once we understand the system. It's very easy for me to see a situation through the eyes of others.	You will find me strident in my lack of stridency. I may poke fun at extreme points of view but I'll respect the "good" parts of the message.

Table 1 My Personality Quirks

For much of my life, I bounced between being overweight and underweight. However I have never been fitter, stronger, and healthier than I am right now, and I've been this way for most of my middle-aged years. I won't spend a lot of time talking about the specifics of how I made this happen because this is your story, not mine. And while many of the techniques are the same, the details of the plan should be custom developed for you. Just know that leading a healthy lifestyle did not come naturally to me. I am not athletic or even coordinated. And I've always been surrounded by bad influences when it came to my own health. Fortunately, you'll find everything you need to know to develop a plan within these pages. The resulting plan allows you to work around your unique environment and tastes.

Professionally, I have over thirty years' experience in the high tech products sector. I am co-inventor of two patents focused on clinical data management that served as the springboard for a machine learning and medical informatics startup. This put me in the position to examine much of our healthcare delivery process from behind the scenes. Between that experience and my unnatural, irrational and insatiable curiosity about physical health, mental health, and physiology, I decided to get involved on the front lines. As a result, I earned my certification as an Exercise Nutritionist and am a trained Integrative Health Coach. I currently operate a health coaching business called Live Long Lead Long (livelongleadlong.com) and have clients from all walks of life who share the trait of being overscheduled and overstressed.

This Book's Origin Story
The Karma Sense Eating Plan emerged from one of those wild dreams I occasionally get that shakes me awake in the middle of the night and prevents me from falling back to sleep as my mind races. When this occurs, I usually get up, jot down a few notes, and that clears my head enough so I can catch a few more Zzzzs. Often when I wake up the next day, I realize that whatever I thought was genius the night before is actually the most stupid freaking idea I've ever heard and toss it. Not this time. When I woke up the next day I felt like I was on to something;

a way of life that is inclusive, healthful and spreads happiness and good will.

I knew I was on the right track and spent much of the next day researching and writing. That night we ate Chinese takeout for dinner and I found this in my fortune cookie:

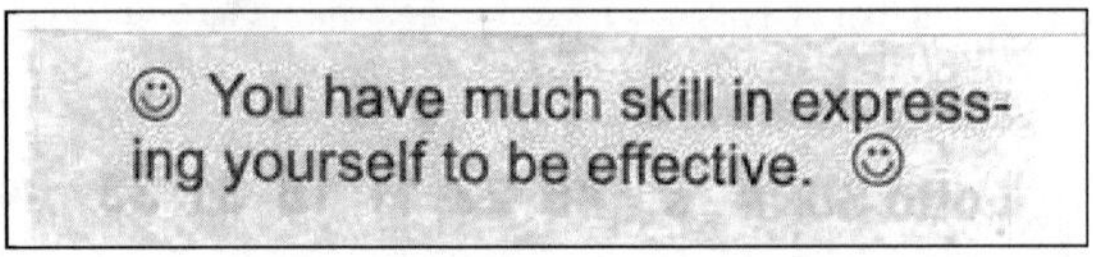

☺ You have much skill in expressing yourself to be effective. ☺

Figure 3 My Favorite of the Received Fortunes[14]

I posted this fortune on Facebook and several friends who had read my blog remarked that this was kismet (kismet is the lazy person's karma. It depends on fate while karma depends on action). Or was it irony? Irony occurs when the literal meaning of something is the opposite of the intended meaning. Such a poorly worded compliment on my communication skills would certainly qualify as irony.

But then I started blogging about the plan. I was really pleased to see how many people read that first post. And the second one reached even more people. But as I got deeper into the subject, it became obvious that a book would be a better format for *The Karma Sense Eating Plan* than a series of blog posts. While working on the book, I continued blogging about it so I wouldn't leave the existing readers hanging.

What this means is everything you need to know about living a life of Karma Sense is out there on the blog for free. If you're reading this book, you either:

1. Appreciate the concept, recognize its value, and decided to invest in your health, happiness, and world saving abilities by purchasing this book; or
2. Somehow got a free copy. No questions asked, just remember that all profits go to charity. If you didn't pay, feel free to directly

donate the value of this book to charity. You don't need me to do it for you; or

3. Are smacking yourself in the head because you dropped a few bucks on this thing when you could have gotten the gist of it for free on the internet.

Regardless of which is true, I thank you for taking the time to read this.

But why don't I stop talking about what you're about to read and actually let you get down to reading it?

The *Karma Sense Eating Plan* Overview

Executive Summary

I'm a happy, healthy person. I made my way into the health and wellness field because I want to help others be healthy and happy as well. I want them to do so without worrying about nutrition dogma and hype. My goal is to get the word out to as many people as possible that being healthy is not an all-or-nothing proposition and that small steps often lead to giant leaps. I recognize that to achieve all this; I have to demonstrate my expertise.

But being an expert comes with baggage. You have to differentiate yourself to be heard over the pabulum from the media, other experts, and companies pushing products. I've listed some examples below of attempts to influence our health decisions based on incomplete information or flat out attempts at deception.

- An article about the dangers of eating kale in *Craftsmanship* magazine goes viral even though the person making the claim is not a scientist, and the claim is not based on any actual research.[15]
- The self-proclaimed "Food Babe" targeted the Subway food chain for adding a "yoga mat material" as an ingredient in its bread.[16] It's true, Subway did add azodicarbonamide to its bread but so do over 500 other food companies.[17] It's a food additive used to whiten flour and condition dough and it's approved by the Food and Drug Administration (FDA). If we're worried about yoga mats and bread containing azodicarbonamide, why aren't we also worried about the fact that both contain dihydrogen monoxide (a.k.a., water)? I'm not saying azodicarbonamide is the equivalent of water. Personally, I avoid azodicarbonamide but not because it's dangerous. I avoid it because I don't need it and I don't care if my bread is chewy and some color other than white.

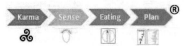

- A popular diet by Dr. William Davis, _Wheat Belly_, implores followers to eat grain-free because of multiple evils and dangers. Grains do not play an essential role in our diets and avoiding them may help people lose weight, but grains are not harmful to most people and have positive benefits when eaten in moderation.[18]

- Another fad diet, _The Bulletproof Diet_, by Dave Asprey, a technology executive (nothing wrong with that!) with no nutrition background, guides followers to have a breakfast consisting only of coffee (preferably "Bulletproof" brand), butter, and other added fats. The purported health benefits of this breakfast are endless, according to Asprey. For most people, there is nothing wrong with skipping breakfast, drinking coffee, and consuming fat. But there is no magic in it either and, for some, it can be unhealthful.[19]

Now, I find myself at a crossroads. Based on the above, if I want to be taken seriously, I need a sticky meme or catchy plan to call my own. On one hand, I do want to be taken seriously. On the other hand, I know that in the best case, these diets and claims are nothing new (worst case, they're utter nonsense). The laws of biology, physics, chemistry and math never change no matter how much butter you put in your coffee.

So because of this internal conflict, I created _The Karma Sense Eating Plan_. It's a plan that supports people who want to be healthier, happier and, oh yeah, save the world. It's a plan that acknowledges the basic and common truths about achieving that happy, healthy state. And it's a plan that does not require objectionable foods and unrealistic habits to work. Sound too good to be true? I'm going to spend the rest of this book demonstrating that nothing could be more true, but first, the name.

Karma

I'm a big believer in karma. You may be telling yourself, "Self, an evidence-based approach to wellness is a key tenet of _The Karma Sense_

Eating Plan. In the Executive Summary of this very chapter, the so-called author refers to laws of science. How could this 'author' possibly believe in karma?"

Well, I'm glad you asked. It's a common expression that nice guys finish last.[20,21] The implication of this expression is that not-so-nice guys finish first (or at least better than last). The implication is wrong. When people cheat, take short cuts, or move in their own interests at the expense of everyone else, they tend to get what they want in the short-term. But in the process, they lose good will, and they delude themselves into thinking that selfishness gets them what they want. So the next time they push even further, and the folks who got burned last time are now looking out for it. At some point, their acceptance of risky behavior exceeds the trust they once had. SNAP! They're busted! I call this the *A-Hole Inflection Point*.

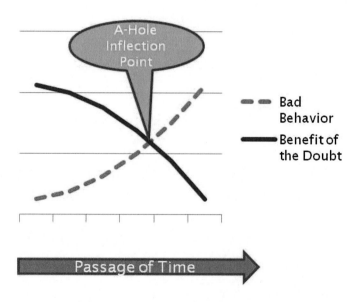

Figure 4 The A-Hole Inflection Point[22]

Meanwhile, people who look out for the interest of others create a different effect. They get to operate within a zone of trust and support that has their back, even after they occasionally stumble because no one's

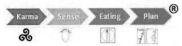

perfect. Adam Grant covers the subject of givers vs. takers more eloquently and in depth in his book, *Give and Take: Why Helping Others Drives Our Success.*[23]

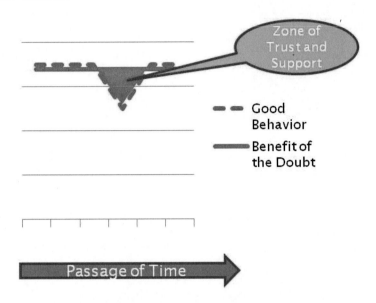

Figure 5 The Zone of Trust and Support[24]

The saying should not be "Nice guys finish last." It should be "Nice guys finish, period." Or to repeat a quote attributed to Chalene Johnson, *"You are the one who teaches other people how to treat you. What do you teach?"* [25,26]

Unfortunately, despite pithy quotes and even Adam Grant's book, limited research exists regarding karma. I had more success finding studies by people named "Karma" than I had on the subject of karma. However, karma is real, and as soon as I find an institution to fund my research on the topic (with you as the potential subject), we'll have evidence.

But what does any of this have to do with an eating plan? I'll tell you as you get deeper into this book. For the purposes of this overview, I hope you agree that, if we can build some nice guy and gal habits into our eating, into something we do all the time, our lives will become a regular party. Because as Abraham Lincoln famously said in the documentary film, *Bill and Ted's Excellent Adventure*, "Be excellent to each other and party on, dudes!"

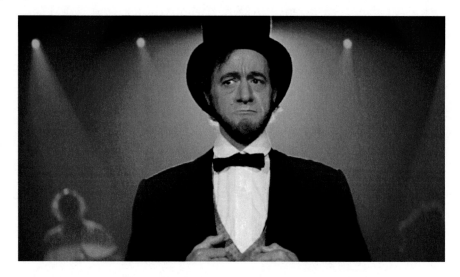

Figure 6 "Be excellent to each other and party on, dudes!"[27,28]

Sense

As it relates to *The Karma Sense Eating Plan*, the term *Sense* has a double meaning

Sense as in Common Sense

Regardless of whether you're trying to lose fat, gain muscle, feel more energetic or just achieve optimal health, the basic facts of good nutrition remain constant. Nothing changes these facts. Not gluten. Not fat. Not sugar. Not eating raw food. Not eating like a modern Asian, ancient Greek, or Fred Flintstone.

I chose PN for my nutrition certification because they're well-respected in the health and fitness community, evidence-based, accessible to full-time workers, and don't try to represent themselves as something they aren't (I'll mention no names. You certificate mills know who you are!). PN presents three styles of eating to its coaches. At one extreme is a highly flexible approach that promotes eating different food groups

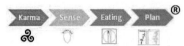

according to specific ratios. At the other extreme is a rigorous plan that includes a daily calorie limit and imposes an exact number of grams per day for each macronutrient (protein, carbohydrates, and fat). The third style falls in the middle.

In reality, each is a different version of exactly the same thing; managing food intake, managing calories, and managing macronutrients. They differ only in how much leeway they provide. As a coach, I choose among the plans depending on client goals, motivation, commitment, knowledge, and results. *The Karma Sense Eating Plan* also has three-ish levels tied to how specific your goals are, your level of knowledge, and your motivation. I'll discuss these more when I describe the Plan component.

Sense as in Feeling

I'm no expert in mindfulness or its sub-genre, mindful eating, but like most aspects of mindfulness, it's highly personal. There are experts who can guide you through specific implementations of mindfulness but regardless of your approach, the end justifies the means. I've been following various flavors of mindfulness for years and never knew it. I just referred to what I was doing as "doing nothing," as in "Dear, I'm going into my office to do nothing so I'd appreciate a little quiet." With these disclaimers aside, there are three aspects of *The Karma Sense Eating Plan* rooted in the act of eating mindfully.

- **Aforementioned Karma** — The plan pairs your eating with intentional (as opposed to random) acts of kindness. By joining the two, you break out of the ingrained habits of your current eating patterns. If you're thinking "How will I help improve the world today as I eat my <insert what you're eating here, but not literally here because it will make this page messy>" you're rewiring your brain to look at eating in a completely different way. And we naturally look at things that are new and different with a lot more curiosity, introspection, and care. This results in more conscious consumption of the amount and quality of our food.

- **Moment of Gratitude** — Unlike with karma, the <u>research</u> on gratitude is solid.[29] Expressing gratitude in some tangible way makes a person more optimistic, happier, healthier, more creative, and more intelligent. Furthermore, as with karma, linking a new practice to something that you usually do without thinking will make you start thinking again. We can express gratitude in many ways ranging from prayer to simple acknowledgment of the people who make, prepare, and serve our food.

- **Eat Slowly and Stop Before You're Full** — Pardon? This is certainly a departure from the two lofty predecessors. From touchy-feely karma and gratitude to this specific and measurable directive? Well yeah, it's specific and measureable but it's also a difficult concept to master. What is "slowly"? How do I know I'm not full when it takes twenty minutes for my body to feel satiated? Exactly! Here we're working with the mind-body connection. It's a discussion that requires an entire chapter on its own. So I don't leave you hanging, here's a question. Do you take less than twenty minutes to eat breakfast, lunch, or dinner? If so, you're probably not eating slowly.

So Sense has these dual actions of applying logic and fact to your eating while getting in touch with your feelings. *The Karma Sense Eating Plan* has something for right brainers and left brainers. That's why it's not Common Sense; It's Karma Sense.

Eating

For the Eating component, I describe what, when, why, and how you should eat. It's the meat-and-potatoes of the plan. But don't worry, both meat AND potatoes are gluten-free and contain no yoga mat material.

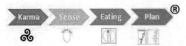

When it comes to the what, when, why and how of eating, the plan asks you to adopt these five habits:

1. Eat Slowly and Stop Before You're Full
2. Eat Protein in Every Meal
3. Eat More Vegetables and Fruits
4. Eat Whole Food Carbohydrates After Vigorous Exercise
5. Eat Good Fats Daily and Balance a Variety of Good Fats

These habits are the mantras of *The Karma Sense Eating Plan*. They also fully meet the nutritional needs and goals of the average person. But who among us is average? People have allergies. People have aversions to certain foods. People have physiological challenges (e.g., diseases that may affect how they should eat). Some people are trying to lose fat, some are looking to maintain, and some want to gain weight (often muscle). All of these introduce subtle and not-so-subtle exceptions to the above. For example, people who are looking to gain weight may need to modify mantra #1. If they want the weight to become muscle they'll have to include exercise whereas, to lose weight, exercise is encouraged but optional. The variables that make us unique drive future discussions in this book about how to adjust these rules.

As with anything that may look like a diet, one of the biggest issues people have is sticking to it. *The Karma Sense Eating Plan* does not expect 100% compliance. In fact, there is an expectation that you will not comply. Cheat days, refeeds, noncompliance, or whatever you want to call it, with this plan, there will be times when you let your hair down and do what you please. How often and when this occurs depends on your goals.

Plan

Admittedly I struggled before adding the word Plan to the end of *Karma Sense Eating*. The obvious choice would be *Diet*, but I dislike the word when attached to a style of eating. To me it has a connotation of being restrictive and temporary. This plan is neither of these things. It's inclusive and you can honor it for the rest of your life.

Diet also implies that we're only talking about eating. The plan's *Karma* component is about doing something good for others. This could be related to eating, but it doesn't have to be. You can choose.

So I landed on *Plan*. And when you reach the description of the *Plan* component, I think you'll agree this is the best term. Between the narrative in that chapter and the tools provided in the appendices, *The Karma Sense Eating Plan* provides everything you need to develop your individual roadmap for improved health, happiness and making the world a better place.

When you put all this together, you get—

The Karma Sense Eating Plan

The Karma Sense Eating Plan describes how to achieve the healthiest and happiest version of you using a modular *plug-and-play* approach. Anyone can adopt this nutrition style to become healthier, happier and, oh yeah, save the world. Anyone! Carnivore, Omnivore, Herbivore, Locavore (not to be confused with locovore which I think is what you call people who eat crazy stuff), Anyone! It works as well for the frugal as it does for the lavish. It can be adopted little-by-little or all at once. In part or in whole. Regardless, you will reap the benefits.

Adopting any one of the plan's components will lead towards greater health and happiness. Put them all together and you're taking a big step towards saving the world.

The sections and chapters that follow describe all of the components and mantras in depth.

Karma

Karma: The Best Way to Start Your Day

Executive Summary

This chapter describes the role that karma plays in your quest for better health and happiness. It explains why good karma is a worthy pursuit regardless of whether you believe it exists. Finally, it provides practical suggestions about how to honor this aspect of the plan.

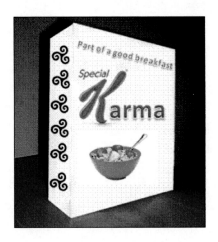

Figure 7 Part of a Complete Breakfast[30]

The Case for Karma

Karma is a tough subject for someone like me. As I said in my Origin Story, I've never been good at jumping to conclusions or trusting my gut. Because I operate this way, I looked for real data on the phenomenon while developing this plan and didn't find much.

Here is what I discovered. In a recent study, scientists looked at teacher assessments of kindergarten students and their ability to get along with others (e.g., sharing, helping, etc.).[31] They compared that information to how well the kids performed academically and socially thirteen to nineteen years later. The researchers found that being nice in kindergarten was a strong predictor of future success.

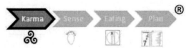

In another study, researchers rated the narcissism of leaders of public companies and established that bombastic CEOs did not perform any better or worse than their more modest peers.[32] While this isn't a ringing endorsement for "Nice guys finish last" it doesn't prove the opposite either. It simply implies that there are many factors at play and you don't need to be a selfish jerk to succeed.

There are some popular books that examine the subject and take various positions. There's the aforementioned *Give and Take: Why Helping Others Drives Our Success*. Also on the side of "good wins," is *The Power of Nice: How to Conquer the Business World with Kindness.*[33] Taking the opposing view, there's *The Upside of Your Dark Side: Why Being Your Whole Self--Not Just Your "Good" Self--Drives Success and Fulfillment.*[34] But none of these objectively shows whether the light side or the dark side reigns when it comes to getting ahead. In the end, they depend upon anecdotes to prove their points.

Well if the best we have are anecdotes, I may as well resort to my own experience. It's based on long-term observation (because I'm old and can observe things over the long-term). Through that observation, I've seen that people who do the right thing most often outperform people who don't. I'm not talking about perfect angels. I'm talking about people who are generally concerned about the welfare of others.

And because of this, I am a full-out believer. However, despite the fact that this chapter promotes karma, I'm not going to make a case that karma is real. You either believe, or you don't. For every example I come up with to prove my point, someone will come up with an example proving the opposite. It's too subjective. The nice thing about karma, as it relates to this plan, is that you don't have to believe in it to experience the benefit.

If you're someone who wants to do the right thing, wants to be a good person, and cares about other people, what I am about to propose will help get you what you want. If you're only interested in your own health and happiness, what I am about to propose will also help get you what you want. Welcome to the win-win scenario

What I Am About to Propose

No doubt you always try to be nice, helpful, polite, and kind. But there may be a little more you could do, right? I propose that you start by doing one additional intentionally nice thing per day. Try to associate this nice act with a meal, and try to smile to yourself about it immediately before the meal. Not only will you make someone happy, but by associating the action with a meal, you will consciously recognize that you are about to eat food. You will recognize that what you are about to eat is special because it is related to someone else's happiness. You will treat that meal differently from the way you treat most meals. That difference will make you more mindful. Because you are more mindful, you will find it easier to consciously eat more slowly and recognize when you're satisfied but not full (an important part of the Sense and Eating components I'll discuss later). And, because you consciously eat more slowly and recognize when you're satisfied but not full, you'll eat healthier. Eating healthy is a key benefit and goal of the plan.

Although we're striving for flexibility with *The Karma Sense Eating Plan*, there are always a few guidelines. Here are the guidelines for the Karma component.

1. When preparing to eat, or soon after, do something nice that you wouldn't normally do. If you usually wash the dishes after dinner, then I'm afraid that doesn't count. There is an infinite number of kind things you can do. I'll even throw out some examples in just a bit. Try something new. It's great if your act of kindness is food or meal-related. This will make it easier to create the associations that are part of the plan. But like everything else in the plan, there's plenty of latitude.

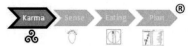

2. If you adopt a good karma practice, and it becomes a habit, refer to #1 above. Add something new so you can continue to expand your good karma portfolio. People say it takes twenty-one days for something to become a habit or to break a habit. Research does not support this. But if it helps to have a goal, pick a number between twenty-one and sixty and go with that. Making this a habit is not a requirement. But if you do, mix things up a little by adding a new one.

3. Although starting one new karma practice a day is a great idea, try to adopt a new one with each meal and see how many you can add. Being kind doesn't necessarily take extra time.

Good Karma Options

Here is a small sample of things you can do. What makes the Karma component so awesome is that it respects your personal definition of kindness. It doesn't impose some new or alien moral code upon you. The only requirement is that your choice be an act of kindness you don't normally do.

#	Karma Act	Comment
1	Cook a meal for someone.	Is there any better meal-related kindness?
2	Buy food from a local source.	Supports local business and the traditional vs. factory farm.
3	Instead of throwing out food waste, use 100% of a food.	Example: use meat or vegetable scraps to make stock or to create an interesting article of clothing.
4	Share *The Karma Sense Eating Plan* with friends who you believe would be interested.	The network effect of good karma. A kindness to me.
5	Clean up after a meal.	To experience the plan's true effect, acknowledge you'll do this before beginning your meal.

#	Karma Act	Comment
6	Eat a smaller meal than usual, and donate the money you save to charity.	A win-win scenario if you want to lose weight.
7	Walk to buy your food or meal.	A win-win-win scenario to improve the environment, traffic, and physical activity.
8	Give a server an extra tip.	The server depends on that income and isn't paid enough for what he or she has to put up with.
9	Thank the restaurant staff who cooked and served you in a very personal and specific way.	They're working their tails off. In addition to tipping, this means a lot to them.
10	Help someone who has trouble eating no matter their reason.	Just do so in a way that maintains dignity.
11	Offer to engage a health coach to help an eating companion with health concerns.	Do so in a loving way. Respect your companion's autonomy and readiness to change.
12	Eat cruelty-free food.	Does not harm animals or other humans in a cruel or unusual way.
13	Tolerate/accept any annoying meal related habit which your eating companion engages in.	If it isn't hurting anyone, let it be.
14	Stop a meal related habit you know annoys your eating companion.	Even if it's harmless, do it as an act of love.
15	Agree to give a loved one 100% of your attention before, during, and/or after a meal.	For example, a discussion or some other kind of favor for the person.
16	Post other ideas on the blog post where this first appeared, on the Live Long Lead Long Facebook page, or send me a tweet with #KarmaSense that associate acts of kindness to eating.	The network effect of good Karma. A kindness to other readers.

Table 2 Karma Ideas

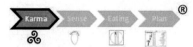

Remember, while you'll be performing these acts of kindness out of the goodness of your heart, there is a selfish reason you're doing this as well.* We're trying to shake up your eating routine so you treat mealtime in a way that will ultimately drive better health. If you take on a karma project that does not occur immediately before eating (e.g., shopping, tipping, cleaning, etc.), find a way to acknowledge the act just before digging in. If this sounds complicated, don't worry about it now. We'll talk about how to deal with this challenge in more detail when we discuss the Sense component.

For now, there are a few things you can do. The right thing for you depends on what is running through your mind as you're reading this.

If what you're saying to yourself sounds like this (group 1):

"I'd like to do this Karma Sense thing, but I know me. I can't suddenly change what I have done for years no matter how good an idea this is. I'll simply never remember to do all this without help. But ol' Davey H's writing style is a true abomination. It will take me a long time to recover from the trauma of reading this far. I won't be able to pick this book up again for at least a month."

Take on the partial adoption approach. Just try to do a new (to you) karma appropriate act of kindness every day and don't worry about the rest. You will be well on your way to being Karma Sensible by the time you read the next few chapters.

If what you're saying to yourself sounds something like this (group 2):

"The jury is out. I would like to live a healthier, happier lifestyle and save the world in one fell swoop, but I'm not convinced this will help. However, what I've read so far is not quite as painful as a root canal, so I will see how it plays out and decide what to do once I read more."

---

* There is nothing wrong with being selfish. Our very existence is often a kindness to someone else.

I'd still recommend the partial adoption approach. Just defer doing anything Karma Sense related until your skeptical mind is satisfied.

If, however, what you're saying to yourself sounds something like this (group 3):

"This is the most ridiculous pile of drivel I've ever seen. We are all stupider for having read this. Yet, much like any train wreck, I am oddly drawn to it. At the very least, it will supply an endless opportunity to troll."

I recommend that you bring on your best trolling. I relish the opportunity to go tête-à-tête (which I believe is French for mano a mano).

The point is (which group 1 people wish I said to begin with), I don't recommend that most people attempt to go all Big Bang over *The Karma Sense Eating Plan*. This likely won't work. Instead, bite off as much as you can chew in one swallow. (See what I did there?) As this book draws to its exciting conclusion, we'll talk about more specific implementation strategies.

In case you weren't taking notes, here's a recap.

Key Points
1. You don't have to believe in karma to reap the plan's benefits.
2. To adopt the Karma Sense style of eating, choose a new act of kindness to associate with a meal and perform this act. It should be something you don't usually do.
3. It would be great if you actually make a habit of your new kind act. If you do, try to add another one to your repertoire (repertoire is French for "stuff that you do").
4. Your ultimate target should be one kind act with each meal. Since these can add up time-wise, you can stop worrying about key point #3 when you get to this stage.
5. If your kind act is something that can't be timed to occur immediately before you begin eating, take the time to consciously

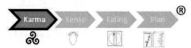

acknowledge it. This will make sure you are conforming to the Sense component, something I'll discuss in a later chapter.

Karma Sense in the Wild

An early adopter of *The Karma Sense Eating Plan* from my original blog series told me that his daughter asked him to drive her to the mall after dinner. This was not something he usually would do but, for the sake of giving the Karma Sense thing a test ride, he agreed. While his daughter shopped, he killed time by walking around to add a few thousand steps on his FitBit. He ended up running into a former colleague, a person whose company he'd always enjoyed, and had a good talk.

In summary:

- Daughter happy – we will discuss the positive health benefits of one's own bliss further in the book. How do you imagine her happiness may have spread? It's the network effect of good karma.
- Exercise goal advanced.
- Personal contact reinforced – the research on the positive health effects of maintaining personal relationships is vast.[35] Assuming that the former colleague felt the same way about the chance meeting (and I do because the person who related this story is a real Mensch, which I believe is French for "cool dude"), the network effect of good karma would be in play again.

All of this with one simple word to a person he loves, "yes."

Save the World? Feh!*

Executive Summary

Throughout this book, I provide research-backed evidence that the Karma Sense lifestyle will make you happier and healthier. But I've gone out on a limb with this "Save the World" thing. What does it even mean? How is it possible if people share different views of what a saved world is? This chapter builds a model for how to deal with this situation so that our varied concepts for a better world can be addressed.

The Save the World Model

Face it, for some people, the world revolves around them. Some people tend to focus on others. And there are people in the middle. As a framework for the discussion in this chapter, the following list encompasses everything that might pertain to a person's view of the world:

- You – Assuming no one is reading over your shoulder and you're not involved in a Karma Sense Eating Plan responsive reading program (because there's no such thing), "You" means the entire corporeal instance of the reader as well as that person's spirit.
- Your Loved Ones – These are the people most important to You.
- The Population at Large – This is all people.
- Other Sentient Beings – This has a specific meaning in Buddhism that I don't even understand. For our purposes, this means all other living creatures with nervous systems, including mammals, fish, birds, reptiles and insects. Since many of these creatures depend on things like plants and single celled entities to live, you can include those too or move them into-
- The Planet – This is everything else that encompasses your world view.

---

* Feh!-An exclamation we will revisit later.

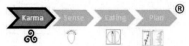

Moving from the top of the list down, each item can be considered a subset of the item below so that graphically you may get something like this.

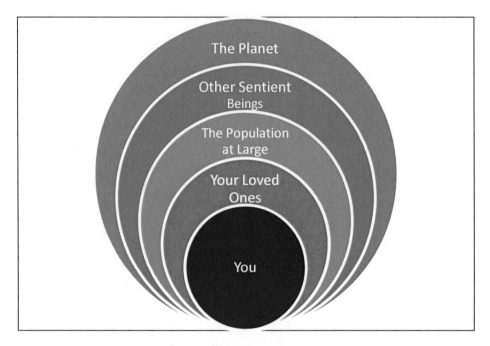

Figure 8 The Save the World Model - All Things Being Equal.[36]

Now suppose you're concerned about each of the items on the list in equal amounts. In other words, if something good happens to you, you perceive it as positively as if something equally good happened to all the creatures on the earth. The model may look like what you see in Figure 8 The Save the World Model - All Things Being Equal.

On the other hand, if all that matters to you are your family, the creatures that inhabit the earth, and the earth itself, you will come up with a figure that looks more like Figure 9 The Save the World Model - A Selfless Person Who Believes Most People Need to Fend for Themselves.

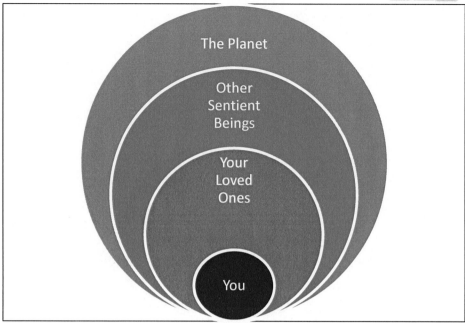

Figure 9 The Save the World Model - A Selfless Person Who Believes Most People Need to Fend for Themselves.[37]

Note that, in this version of the Save the World Model, the You circle is very small compared to the others. Furthermore, The Population at Large is not represented. This is a perfectly legitimate view. You might know someone willing to sacrifice for his or her family and the well-being of stray puppy dogs and mistreated farm animals, but who think other people have the power to stick up for themselves. I don't view things this way, but I don't quarrel with people who do.

An extreme example is someone who is 100% selfish. That model would look like Figure 10 The Save the World Model - A Completely Selfish Person.

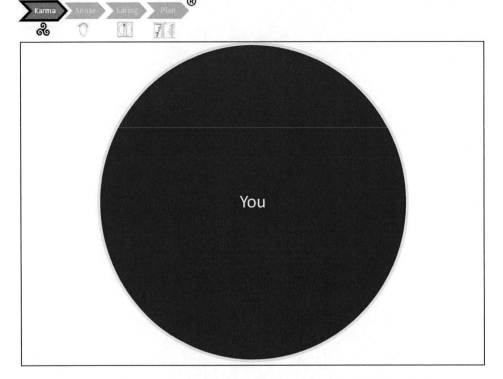

Figure 10 The Save the World Model - A Completely Selfish Person.[38]

I don't believe that anyone like this truly exists nor do I think that such a person would ever read a book with "Karma" in the title, but for the sake of being complete, I needed to represent this situation.

You're Losing Me Here

Sorry about that. Throughout this book, I claim that adopting *The Karma Sense Eating Plan* will save the world. I am not expecting too many arguments about the Karma component. Anyone wanting to argue that a massive movement of people helping others will destroy the world is most likely trolling.

There are other places in the book, specifically with mantra #3, Eat More Vegetables and Fruits, where the save the world claim might not be as obvious. This chapter prepares you for that discussion. But the Save the World Model is also worth referencing any time I claim the plan helps save the world.

Key Points

1. This book assumes that different people place different priorities on what is important, and this affects their vision of what saving the world looks like.

2. This view consists of You, Your Loved Ones, The Population at Large, Other Sentient Beings, and The Planet. The earlier items in the list are a subset of the latter items on the list.

3. Different people will place different priorities on each of these items. There is nothing wrong with that. We don't judge.

4. The Save the World Model becomes relevant again as we explore other aspects of *The Karma Sense Eating Plan* when if offers an opportunity to save the world.

Sense

Common Sense + Sensitivity = Karma Sense

Executive Summary

This chapter covers the theory of how linking your karma-worthy good deeds to a more healthful eating routine leads to greater health and happiness. The cool thing about *The Karma Sense Eating Plan*, if I do say so myself (which I apparently do because I just did), is that it is so inclusive. It doesn't matter what your favorite foods are. How many meals you eat. Breakfast eater or breakfast hater. Republican or Democrat. It combines the rigors of fact, structure, logic, and analysis with the less tangible je ne sais quoi (which I believe is French for "huh?"). It is that yin and yang of the word "Sense" that I discuss here. We start with some high falutin folderol (which is geezer speak for trifle) and follow that up in the next chapter with a discussion on geezers. But more importantly we talk about the practical aspects of how to make this important link.

The Case for (Common) Sense

There are so many variables that impact your health:

- Genetics
- Physiology
- State of Mind
- Physical Activity
- That swerving car up ahead with the Maryland plates (I pick on Maryland but drivers from other states get my goat too. Maybe that's what I get for tooling around I-93 with a goat. But I digress.)
- Nutrition

The Karma Sense Eating Plan primarily focuses on Nutrition (though it does give that State of Mind thing a run for its money too).

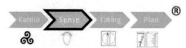

Does the world really need another person to weigh in on how to eat more healthfully? Probably not. Especially because, when you boil it down, there are very few options at play. And like all things that have a finite set of options, I like to summarize them in a table. Wheee!

Goal	Nutrition Solution	Exercise Required?	What Can Help?
Lose Fat	Consume fewer calories than burned	No but highly recommended	*The Karma Sense Eating Plan*
Maintain Weight But Be Healthy	Consume and burn equal # of calories	No but highly recommended	*The Karma Sense Eating Plan*
Gain Weight & Build Muscle	Consume more calories than burned	Yes	*The Karma Sense Eating Plan*
Satisfy Your Own Insatiable Hunger for More Nutrition Information	N/A	N/A	As one of your tribe, I can tell you there is no help for you.

Table 3 Health Goals and Solutions

If you're still patiently reading this book, I assume it's because you have a goal that fits one of the categories in the "Goal" column. If so, the way to reach your goal involves combining what's in the *Nutrition Solution* column and what's in the *Exercise Required?* column. This magical table is the "Cliffs Notes" version of every diet book ever written. (For those of you who don't know what "Cliffs Notes" are, it's what your parents used instead of Wikipedia. In fact, you can learn more about them on Wikipedia).

I admit the last column is a shameless plug (as well as a way to increase my SEO score for the online version). But it also makes an important point about *The Karma Sense Eating Plan*. The plan applies no matter your goal. The plan conforms to the majority of diets you've heard about and maybe even tried. This is what makes *The Karma Sense Eating Plan* so inclusive. It boils all the available hooey about nutrition into the basic irrefutable facts. The plan doesn't denigrate going all raw, juice cleanses, or the marshmallow diet (this diet exists but, while not denigrating it, I refuse to provide further details). Since these styles of eating can coexist with the plan, if they work for you, you're on your way to good health. Also, you'll be helping to save the world. Never forget that minor point.

I'm not claiming that you should implement The Karma Sense Eating Plan in *exactly* the same way regardless of your goal. That would be a lie and therefore not very karma worthy. On one hand, if you want to lose weight, it's possible to do so simply by following the previously discussed mantras (that I'll repeat in lurid detail later). But for many folks, more information and support is required. If, on the other hand, you just want to maintain where you are with an eye towards better health, you're probably fine following the five mantras as-is, provided you carefully watch mantra #1 which urges you to *Stop eating before you're full*. But we'll discuss that in more detail later too. And on the other hand (wait, that makes three hands?!?) *Eating Slowly and Stopping Before You're Full* will likely work against you if you're goal is to gain weight. We'd almost definitely drop that mantra from your repertoire if weight gain is your goal. And finally, if you're in the fourth group, a nutrition nerd, I wish you'd take over the keyboard for a while because I'm starting to get carpal tunnel syndrome.

I discuss these subtleties in detail in the chapters about the Eating component. But at this point, what you need to walk away with is this: while eating healthful can be hard, the rules to healthful eating are easy. They are not only easy but they are logical and backed by extensive research. So with this behind us, I'll appeal to your softer side next.

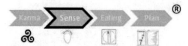

The Case for (Sensual) Sense

Let's depart from cold hard facts (but only a little) and examine the softer side of Sense, the Sensual. To be clear, I don't mean "sensual" in a way that will force me to slap this on the book.

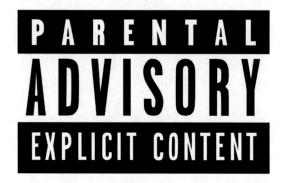

Figure 11 Sensual - The Good Kind

I mean sensual as in "feeling." We'll look at the theory behind how linking acts of karma-kindness to your eating ritual drives healthier habits.

But first, a story.

A Story

When I was in college, I found this awesome job. It involved zipping around campus delivering essential nutrition to students who had an inexplicably strong craving for specific foodstuffs. The arrival of these items brought such joy to their lives that they would often reward me with additional cash over and above what they were required to pay. It was as if their judgment was impaired and they had no sense of the value of a dollar. Also, they giggled a lot.

It was a fantastic opportunity. The only problem was that I had to drive the company vehicle, and that company vehicle was a pickup truck with a manual transmission (a.k.a., a stick shift). Well, this here city feller never drove one of them there manually transmitted vehicles before. Fortunately, this feller was datin' a farmer's granddaughter, and she was well versed in the intricacies of operating such equipment.

So on my first day of work, I picked up the keys from this purveyor of fine vittles and met that there aforementioned country gal at the truck. As I stalled and backfired my way through the streets of Tobacco Road, she was patient and kind and only screamed in horror when absolutely necessary, such as the time I rolled backwards and downhill into some young fraternity man's BMW because I couldn't engage first gear.

Eventually, with hard work and perseverance, this here feller got to the point where driving a manual transmission became second nature. Fortunately there weren't cell phones or Starbucks back then because my expertise graduated to a level that would have allowed me to easily hold a Triple Venti Bacon Caramel Macchiato in one hand, update my Facebook relationship status from "It's Complicated" to "Married" in my other hand, and shift into overdrive with my head tucked in just the right position (because I still deny that I have three hands).

The moral of this story is twofold:

1. If you ever date someone who knows how to drive a truck with a manual transmission, and that person is willing to teach you, he or she is THE ONE. Get married immediately. This act will ensure your eternal happiness.
2. When we first learn a new skill, we pay attention to every detail required to perform the skill. We pay attention in a very deliberate way. Eventually it becomes second nature, and then we do all the detailed steps without thinking about them. Everything good we learned about that skill while we were acquiring it becomes hard-coded in our brains. Everything bad we learned also finds a comfortable home.

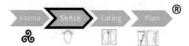

Back to the Point Which I Spent Way Too Much Time Away From, All For the Sake of a Back Story

A scenario similar to my back story happened to you when you were learning how to eat and feed yourself. While you may not have come dangerously close to $10,000 damage to a German sports car, you probably did explore the feeling of strained peas in your ear canal every once in a while. But eventually, the act of eating became second nature. You didn't have to think about it.

There is nothing wrong with that. In fact, it's great when the stuff you have to do to live becomes easy. It happened when you learned to breathe. It happened when you learned to drink water. It happened when you learned to eat. All of these are basic requirements for life.

If you sort these basic requirements in order from most vital for life to least, you get what you see on the horizontal axis of the chart below (by the way, tables are the gateway drug to graphs and charts).

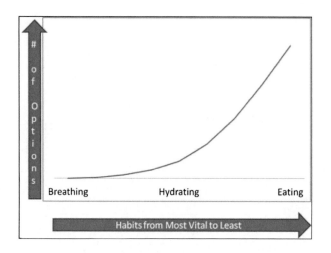

Figure 12 Habits Required to Live and How Easy It Is to Screw Them Up[39]

If you then plot these requirements against the number of options you have for satisfying them, you see that the more vital the activity, the fewer choices you have for completing it. The fewer choices, the harder it is to introduce divergent habits, whether good or bad. Yes, one person can do a better job of breathing than another, but the difference is a hair's breadth. And the way some people drink is totally hilarious, but as long as they're getting hydrated, what's the harm?

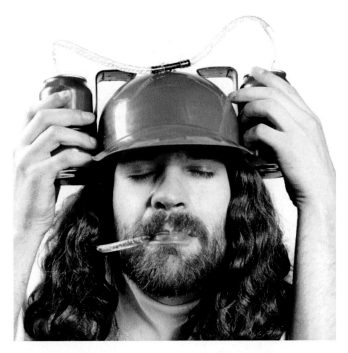

Figure 13 This Feller Has a Drinking Problem[40]

But with a requirement like nourishment, you have tons of ways to introduce undesirable habits that you don't even notice. How do we get you to notice them? Let me tell you about driving a stick shift.

Driving a Stick Shift

At this point in my life, I'm very comfortable driving a stick shift. But what would happen if a sudden change shocked my stick-shift-driving-

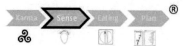

environment? For example, I'm not a fan of snakes. Here is a picture of how I would react to a bunch of snakes:

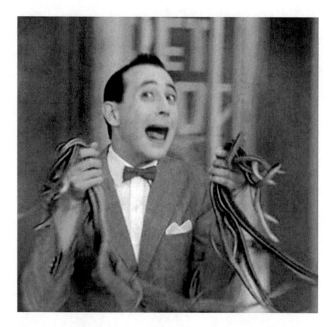

Figure 14 Visual Approximation of Author Reacting to a Bunch of Snakes[41,42]

What if suddenly to change gears in my rockin' 2000 Oldsmobile Alero, I had to reach out and grab a live snake's head? I'd act a lot more considered and deliberate every time I changed gears. And because snakes tend to wriggle and are generally ornery (it's riding in an Oldsmobile Alero, of course it's ornery), I will take a long time to settle into a static habit for changing gears. Suddenly shifting gears goes from being a mind-LESS activity to a mind-FUL activity.

Well fortunately, *The Karma Sense Eating Plan* doesn't involve any snakes (unless you follow the Snake Diet in which case the snake would be part of your protein with every meal). With the plan, we're going to use your act of good karma and one other powerful but simple activity to mess with your mind a little. And this is going to help you find and eject the bad eating habits you developed over time.

But for now, I need to close this chapter because I am exceeding my arbitrary self-imposed word limit. I established a word limit because, unlike in person where I communicate mostly with grunts and rude noises, in writing I tend to go stream-of-consciousness. Of course, I could fix that by removing all the bloviating about the halcyon days of my youth as well as the tables and charts, but those are what make me so darn lovable☺. So I'll continue with the details of Sense in the next chapter.

Key Points

1. No matter your health goal, the nutrition aspects are invariably tied to calories consumed and calories burned. All the plans and diets you've ever heard of depend on this fact.
2. Habits develop over time and are hard to change. To change them, you first have to know you have them.

Sense: Shake It Up Break It Down

Executive Summary

This chapter includes practical suggestions about how to link acts of kindness to the food you eat for the sake of a better you and a better world. And to do that, we're going to have to take a look at your current relationship with food and mealtime, as well as explore an old phenomenon.

Geezer-dom

I admit it, I'm a geezer. But I try hard not to think, act, or pine for the old days like geezers tend to do. For example, when one of my geriatric peers says, "Feh!" (which is a geezer's way of saying "I don't understand, but I want to express general disapproval anyway") and follows his or her "Feh!" with complaints about "kids today" and their video games and their face piercings and how they're all lazy, I usually toss a "geezer" flag.

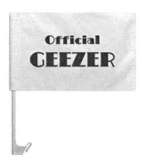

Figure 15 It's Official[43]

And declare a twenty-yard penalty. The twenty yards are good exercise even though it takes the typical geezer much of the day to go that far.

That wasn't such a great example. Here's a better one (at the very least you can't deny that it's a different one). We'll progress through this

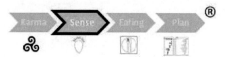

example by simulating one of those BuzzFeed quizzes that are so popular with you kids today (BuzzFeed; yet another thing we geezers ruined.)

With this single-question quiz, we'll predict an important fact about you based on your answer. Here is the question:

When you think of a song with the title "Shake It Up," what performer comes to mind?

A. The Cars
B. Taylor Swift
C. Selena Gomez
D. None of the above

If you picked A, the Cars: You're a geezer

This song is from the 80s. The lyrics consist of little more than "Dance all night" and "Shake it up.[44]" You still can't accept that a more nuanced song could possibly be released by a recent artist.

If you picked B, Taylor Swift: You need to work on your reading comprehension

I said "Shake It Up." not "Shake It Off.[45]" Nice try, though. Catchy.[*]

If you picked C, Selena Gomez: You're a student of behavioral science and the theory of habit change

This song accompanied a short-lived Disney Channel series (that I had no idea existed until I started researching this chapter. Surprised that I actually research this stuff, eh?), and includes these lines taken directly from a textbook on habit change theory (that I should write someday):

Shake it up!
Break it down[46]

---

[*] Shake It Off's lyrics are more appropriate for *The Karma Sense Mindfulness Plan – How to be Save the World by Doing Nothing,* available in 2017.

These two lines contain everything we need to do to reprogram eating habits and to reap the rewards of Karma Sense Eating. With The Karma Sense Eating Plan, we "Shake it up!" by building some new habits to use just before eating. We "Break it down" by slowing down and encouraging you to enjoy your meal in ways you now take for granted.

If you picked D, None of the above: You are not only a geezer but your negative attitude is kind of bringing the rest of us down

You responded this way because either your music appreciation pre-dates the 1980s or you're making a snide remark (a.k.a., snark) and being snarky is also something we geezers ruined for the youth of today. Snark is out. Positivity is in. I know it's in because it's a crucial part of *The Karma Sense Eating Plan*.

With this scholarly review of the theory of habit change as brought to us by Dr. Selena Gomez behind us, let's look at the first step to apply your senses to Karma Sense Eating.

Shake it up!

I'm going to be serious for a minute (well, maybe just a little). "Shake it up" is a very concise but flip way of explaining an important concept in *The Karma Sense Eating Plan*.

Mind-LESS eating is a problem, and Mind-FUL eating is the solution. You eat mindlessly when any of the following occurs:

- You're distracted (eating while watching TV, eating at your desk at work, obsessing over what you should have said to Jenkins when he made that wise-crack two hours ago).
- Binge eating or eating until stuffed.
- Not thoroughly enjoying the eating experience.
- Feeling bad physically or mentally as a result of what you ate.

Mindful eating is a state in which you completely focus on the process of eating. You're experiencing the entire activity with all your senses and

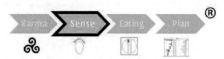

across the dimension of time. When it comes to eating the Karma Sense way, you're going to "Break it down" into its individual components of texture, smell, taste, and so on. Don't worry, though; you're not going to eat mindfully at the expense of enjoying the company of others. Mindful eating is not mutually exclusive with being socially connected at mealtime. Mindful eating will allow you to enjoy your food in ways you haven't experienced since those strained peas were drying in your ear canal when you were a baby. If you love food, there really is no better way to eat.

Mindful eating has other benefits besides making meals more pleasurable. Research shows that distracted eaters consume more food than people who eat without distractions.[47] Another study demonstrates that introducing a mindful eating practice for obese people resulted in weight loss and reduced stress.[48]

Is mindful eating a panacea to the world's ever-increasing obesity problem (and the chronic disease epidemic that accompanies it)? No. However, research indicates that it will help, and since the downside is limited, it's worth a try. Even if you're sold at this point, there's still a problem. This problem is that the firmly entrenched habits you developed over all these years are so darn hard to break. We're all like geezers in that way. I know. When conceiving this plan, I would get halfway through my meal before realizing I forgot the pre-meal ritual. That's why I asked earlier in this book, and will ask again now, that you do the following two things before you start a meal:

- **Perform an act of good karma.** Without beating a dead horse (which would create bad karma), plan on doing a good deed associated with eating. This will put you in the mindset to practice mindful eating. If your good karma act needs to happen well before a meal or has to wait until after, then just incorporate a reflection of what you did or will do when you perform the second pre-meal ritual, gratitude.

- **Include a moment of gratitude.** There is a spiritual aspect to associating gratitude with meal time. Many religions encourage this practice. Unfortunately, because of religious connotations, people shun or even scoff at the practice (Feh!). I consider myself a spiritual person. The plan's whole concept spawned from this aspect of my life. But spirituality is such a private thing that to inflict a specific brand has no place in a concept like this. The plan strives to be inclusive. The good news in the plan's case is that this moment of gratitude is not just a spiritual device, science backs it. Multiple studies (including this one),[49] show that overt expressions of gratitude lead to greater happiness. Furthermore, people who adopt this type of practice require fewer visits to physicians and exercise more often. For a totally entertaining and informative discussion on the science of happiness, gratitude, health, and intelligence, watch this 12 minute Ted Talk by Shawn Achor.[50]

Your Pre-Meal Ritual

Yes, all this goodness exists, but let's not forget the other reason you're engaging in a pre-meal ritual, to "Shake it up!" We want this ritual to raise awareness that you're transitioning into mealtime. The fact that this also makes you happier is just gravy (Mmmmm, gravy). There are no rules as to how to perform this ritual. If you already have a moment of grace, then just incorporate your new Karma Sense topics. If this is new to you, you can do this sitting or standing, in silence or aloud, head bowed and eyes shut, or head up and eyes open. It doesn't matter. Experiment. Give the wave a try, for all I care.

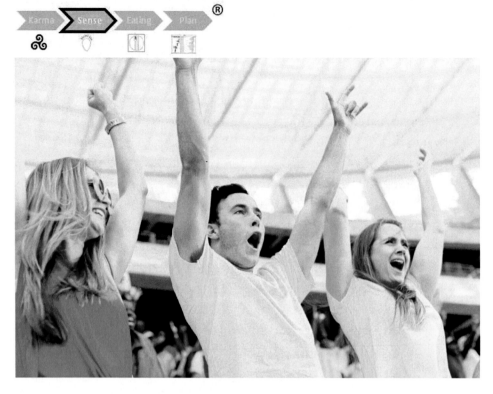

Figure 16 Saving the World is my Goooooaaall![51]

Just include the following in your thoughts.

1. **Your act of good karma.** Think about how it made you feel. How it made the subject of your kindness feel. How it may have spread to others.

2. **A kindness done to you.** Reflect upon something someone did for you that you appreciate. Alternatively, think of a characteristic that someone has that impacted you in a positive way (e.g., Trini always finds the bright side). Whatever you select, think about how it made you feel and how it may have affected others. Consider the variety of ways to thank that person, and commit to one of those ways (e.g., a written thank you, a verbal acknowledgement well after the event occurred). By the way, it's okay if the kindness was done by you and for you. We deserve to pat ourselves on the back now and then.

3. **The actual meal itself**. Consider the fact that everything you are about to eat lived at some point. You extend your life at the expense of another organism's life. You extend others' lives by extending your own (by this I mean other people, creatures, or plants that may depend on you, including the trillions of bacteria living on and in your body). The food you are about to eat lived its life at the expense of some other carbon-based plant or creature (it had to eat too). Another line of thought revolves around the energy required to bring your meal to your table. From the people who grow the food to the people who move the food closer to you. The cooks. The servers. The cleaning crew. And the waste removers. Not to get all *Lion King* on you, but it's the gosh darn circle of life. And it's right there in front of you. It's amazing, beautiful, and delicious all at the same time. Did I mention that food is awesome?

Perhaps the biggest challenge is remembering to perform the ritual in the first place. There are a number of ways you can hack your memory to make this happen. Almost by definition, you already have some kind of ritual (habits!) that you follow before you eat. You drink a glass of water. You lock your computer screen. You set the table. Something. Whatever that thing is, try to disrupt it right now. Move your water glass some-where you don't usually expect it. Change your computer wallpaper. Fold the napkins to look like swans. Do it now. Any of this will start the "Shake it up!" process and remind you to do your pre-meal ritual. My favorite disruptor is to turn on my Spiderman Web Hand.

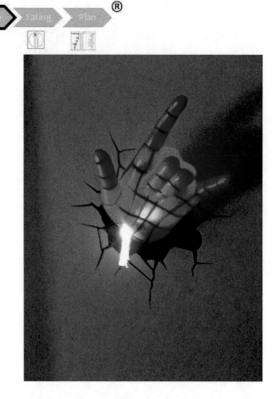

Figure 17 My Spidey Senses Are Tingling[52]

And please, no distractions (look, a squirrel!).

After you enjoy your moment of gratitude (the only way to do this wrong is to not enjoy it), you will be ready to transition to the next phase of Dr. Gomez' program for positive habit development.

Break It Down

If you recall from the plan's Overview chapter, the third element of the Sense component requests that you Eat Slowly and Stop Before You're Full. There are a number of good reasons to do this and many techniques to make it happen in a meaningful and mindful way. To fully reacquaint you with the true pleasure of eating and food, we're going to break the process down into its constituent parts. We'll do that when we get to the Eating component and discuss mantra #1, Eat Slowly and Stop Before You're Full. Eating Slowly and Stopping Before You're Full requires keen attention to how you feel (i.e. your senses). It's also a critical aspect of healthful eating. Therefore, this behavior is relevant to both the Sense and Eating components. It simply can't pick a side. It's wishy-washy in that way. But we love it none the less. And you will learn to love it too, in the next section.

But for now, let's end the discussion on the Sense component with a clarifying chart, because that's how I roll.

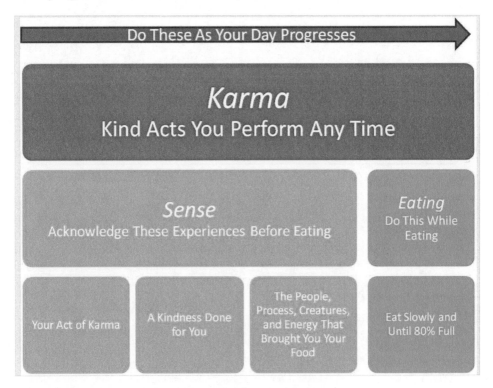

Figure 18 Karma Sense Eating Timeline[53]

Key Points
1. To change deeply ingrained habits, find a way to break your patterns. You need to Shake it up!
2. Shake it up! by introducing a new ritual just before you eat.
3. The ritual should include reflection on a kindness you performed, reflection on a kindness done for you, and acknowledgement of

---

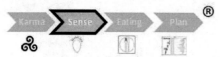

the sacrifice and effort that went into creating your meal. This one act will make you healthier, happier, and wise.

4. This new ritual better positions you for mindful eating. Mindful eating leads to physical, mental, and spiritual well-being.

Karma Sense in the Wild

When first starting my blog, the initial following was small but growing. According to my web statistics, it was also loyal. But I couldn't help feeling like I was talking to empty space because the audience almost never engaged. One reader however, consistently commented and provided me feedback.

That reader is Barbara Greco, a Registered Nurse (RN), a talented artist, an outdoor enthusiast, and an Integrative Health Coach. She's a real Renaissance woman. Recently Barbara sent me a very detailed and complimentary email acknowledging the challenge of creating and publishing *The Karma Sense Eating Plan*. She also expressed her confidence in the eventual success of this project and the positive impact it will have. Her tangible expression of appreciation was out of the blue and came at a perfect time for me. I was feeling overwhelmed by the size of the task. I was in a full out funk. After reading Barbara's note, I realized that nothing had changed from the moment I originally had my "flash of brilliance" except I was much further along in the process. I was much closer to getting it done. Funk be gone!

It struck me, whether she realized it or not, her email represented an example of exactly what the Sense component asks you to do in order to help move you towards greater happiness. I'd like to think that her email was inspired by what she read in *Live Long Lead Long*. So I asked her about it.

I'll let her words speak for themselves.

> "[Some of the things you write about were] *on my mind and I wanted to share it with you. Perhaps subconsciously I was thinking about gratitude because so many of us take things for granted and forget that it's the small stuff that has much meaning and leaves us with hope. It takes courage and dedication to follow through with our dreams. I wrote a brief note because I was touched by some of the sentiments that you wrote. It is not too often that someone is willing to express his feelings…*

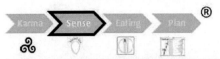

As far as composing the email it felt great...I feel [writing] *lifts peoples spirits and make them feel good. Little gestures go a long way. It can be a simple smile, a friendly hello, a helping hand. I also believe in letting people like you know what a great job they are doing."*

In summary:

- Intentional expressions of appreciation and gratitude can become habit.
- Even after it becomes habit it continues to lift spirits of both the giver and receiver. Barbara and I continue to discuss this phenomenon and each time it's vitalizing.
- Something as easy as dashing off an email of appreciation and gratitude has this spirit-lifting effect.
- It is safe to assume that with both our moods improved, we each engaged with others in a more positive way as well.

Barbara's ability to be positive and grateful is infectious. If you'd like to catch it, you can contact her through her website, bgrecoihc.com.

Eating

A Quick Reintroduction to the Eating Component

The Inclusiveness of the Karma Sense Eating Plan

I keep mentioning that *The Karma Sense Eating Plan* is inclusive. It caters to different tastes, values, and goals. The chapters that follow provide details of the five mantras, summarized here:

1. Eat Slowly and Stop Before You're Full
2. Eat Protein in Every Meal
3. Eat More Vegetables and Fruits
4. Eat Whole Food Carbohydrates After Vigorous Exercise
5. Eat Good Fats Daily and Balance a Variety of Good Fats

Note that these all center on what you *can* do to have a healthful and well-balanced diet. They're not about taking food away or what you *can't* do. The intent is to make sure you get the nutrition you need to thrive physically, emotionally, and spiritually. This means that you can eat with Karma Sense while including whatever foods you crave even if someone else tells you these foods are like what kryptonite is to Superman.

However, this doesn't mean the plan encourages consuming the bad Karma that the food industry inflicts upon us. I personally won't touch stuff with partially hydrogenated anything. I mean, if you need to hydrogenate your stuff, which you don't, finish the job! With the exception of beer and wine, which I can rationalize as healthful in moderation, I won't drink beverages that contain calories or artificial sweeteners. It always shocks my system when I order iced tea in the southeast United States and it comes sweetened by default (I'll never learn). And, I avoid pork because it's so hard for me to find humanely raised hogs. Pigs are probably the most intelligent animals Americans consume. I only eat pork when I can confirm the pigs received humane treatment and sadly, humanely raised hogs are hard to find.

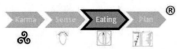

But that's me. You have your own tastes and taboos. If you follow the guidance of the five mantras, you'll maximize your nutrition goodness and still have some room to include your (no-reason-to-feel) guilty pleasures. The plan recognizes that, even though certain foods do not necessarily improve your health, eating them doesn't mean that the occasional transgression will result in an express ride to the Intensive Care Unit.

The human body is a healing machine. In its never ending quest to achieve homeostasis, it fights any foreign invaders that attack it. Whether it's attacked by pollution, bacteria, or bacon-and-ranch-flavored-chocolate-covered-cheese-puffs, the body will prevail as long as we manage and moderate the intake.

It's with this in mind that the plan supports cravings. Even in more managed versions of the plan where you're working with a coach to meet specific goals and timelines, you must respect your tastes. Respecting your autonomy is what this plan is all about. Well, in addition to making you healthier, happier, and oh yeah, saving the world.

The Mantras and Weight Loss

People have many different goals when looking to improve their health. For so many people that goal is to lose weight and *The Karma Source Eating Plan* supports that goal. A limited number of variables exist that affect your weight and body composition. They're in the graph on the next page (Another graph?!? I can feel your eyes rolling from here.).

Moving left to right, you have almost no control over your genes. You have limited power to drive your physiology. Most of that power comes from how well you manage the variables to the right: Physical Activity, Nutrition, and Mindset. The plan does a little to encourage Physical Activity, but not until mantra #4 and even then, barely. It's all about good nutrition and improved mindset.

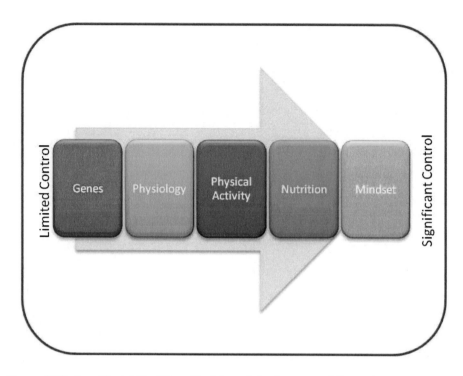

Figure 19 Factors That Affect Your Health and the Amount of Control You Have Over Them[54]

So we have these five things that affect your weight. They seem pretty manageable. But taken together they multiply, divide, and conspire with each other so that one size can never fit all when it comes to losing weight.

I've said before and I'll say again (I know because I've already written the chapter) that the simple equation of eating fewer calories than you burn is the only way to lose weight. Many experts will tell you that it takes a deficit of 3,500 calories spread over time to equal one pound of weight loss. Fortunately, there is a critical mass of other experts who will tell you that this is technically true but meaningless as it applies to any one individual. This is not only because of genes, physiology and so on. All the calorie information you see on food packages and the internet? Those

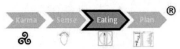

charts that tell you how many calories two hours on the elliptical burns? They're estimates. Estimates that are almost always wrong when applied to a single person.

And then there's this, <u>research</u> shows that for diet adherence, the less complex the rules, the better.[55] I don't fully support this, but I'll get to that shortly. The plan's five mantras are nothing if not simple. They are specifically designed to manage portion size and ensure that you fill up with the most satiating and nutrient-dense foods possible at the expense of eating calorie-dense foods. This alone drives weight loss for many people.

Some people, however, need more support and more complex rules. If the rules are too simple, they're open to interpretation. For example, if you find you're negotiating with the less complex rules of your diet plan (Do bacon-and-ranch-flavored-chocolate-covered-cheese-puffs count as protein? There are two grams in a twelve-ounce bag), that plan is not for you. If, on the other hand, the rules are too complex or too strict, they raise different problems but lead to the same result. Non-adherence.

In summary, *The Karma Sense Eating Plan* stands on its own as a weight loss plan. Some people may want more information, support, and structure. That's fine. There are plenty of resources available to provide that. Let me know if I can help.

The Mantras and Overall Health

I grew up near Exit 10 of the New Jersey Turnpike also known as Edison, New Jersey. At the time its most notable quality was its proximity to where the New Jersey Turnpike crossed the Garden State Parkway (The Crossroads of New Jersey!). Lesser known was the gem shown on the next page.

This 131-foot (forty-meter) tower and accompanying two-room museum stand on the site where Thomas Alva Edison invented the phonograph and perfected the light bulb.

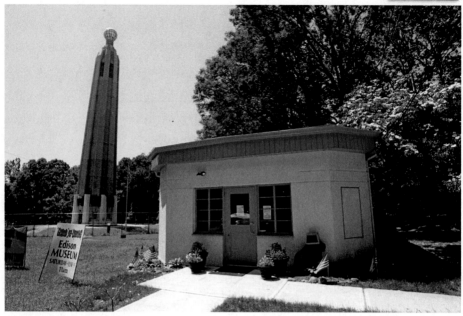

Figure 20 The Mighty Edison Skyline - The Edison Tower and Museum[56]

Thomas Edison was a freethinking polymath. He was a genius inventor and businessman. He was also notoriously difficult to work with. Edison seemed to understand that the modern conveniences he cultivated had a dark side; one that would contribute to our current chronic disease epidemic. As an inventor, his first instinct would have been to create something new to overcome this trend. But why recreate the wheel? Nature already fixed this problem. Here is a prescient comment he made on the future of medicine:

"The doctor of the future will no longer treat the human frame with drugs, but rather will cure and prevent disease with nutrition."--Thomas Alva Edison, 1902-ish[57]

The five mantras of *The Karma Sense Eating Plan* target this exact notion. The research supporting this claim is laid out for you in the descriptions of each. This is not to say that proper nutrition will eliminate the need to seek out "conventional" medicine from time to time. But the two are complementary.

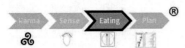

Unfortunately most physicians do not have the nutrition knowledge they should. The National Academy of Sciences recommends a minimum of twenty-five hours of nutrition instruction for medical students. Yet the *average* physician receives less than 80% of that (19.6 hours). Only about a quarter of all doctors ever reach twenty-five hours.[58] When working with your physician to optimize your health, ask questions about the nutritional aspects of any therapy or procedures that your doctor recommends. Also ask for recommendations on resources you can reference on your own time. Doctors who balk at these questions don't deserve to have you as a patient. Either find another or seek supplementary help on your own.

Mantra #1: Eat Slowly and Stop Before You're Full

Executive Summary
This chapter discusses the first mantra of the Eating component. Each of the five Eating mantras has a dedicated chapter. Most of the discussion on Eating delves into the details of specific foods to eat. The first mantra focuses on the *how* and not the *what* of eating. The *how* is Eat Slowly and Stop Before You're Full.

With the housekeeping behind us, there's nothing to do now but discuss Batman.

Batman and the History of How We Eat
In the United States, back before there was MyPlate

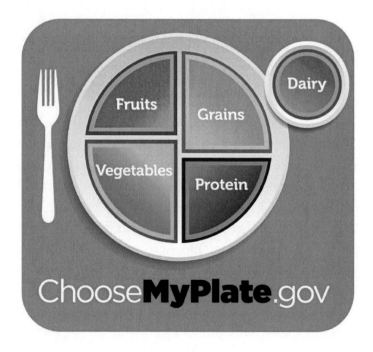

Figure 21 Really? Dairy and Grains a Requirement?[59]

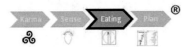
Even before the Food Pyramid,

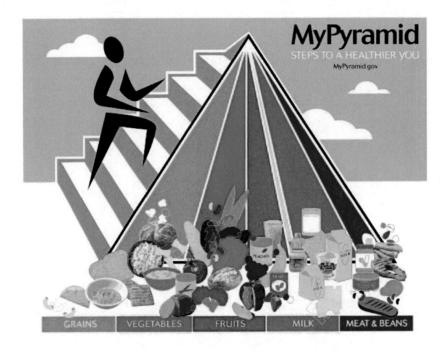

Figure 22 What is This Trying to Say?[60,61]

there were the Basic Four Food Groups (a nutrition guideline that is so embarrassing in its naiveté, it's difficult to find a public domain image for it). Now, we all have our own little jokes for what we consider to be our Basic Four. For the six-year-old version of me, it was hamburgers, ice cream, french fries, and food that seemed better suited as a toy than as something to put in my mouth. Food was more of an edible form of Legos than a source of nourishment. And so, at family meal time, I inevitably was still picking away well after my brother and sister left the table to do whatever adolescents do when they're not eating, sleeping, or primping. The other straggler was my dad, an accomplished slow eater. My dad, Abe Hellman, was unintentionally ahead of his time when it came to personal health. He voluntarily walked miles a day through Manhattan while his colleagues took taxis. Fish was his favorite protein when everyone else was eating steak. He drank alcohol sparingly at a time when the three martini lunch was de rigueur. Mindful eating was just another one of his examples. He didn't know he was being healthy. He just listened to what his body told him to do.

So, with my dad setting the benchmark for the maximum time to complete a meal, if he finished dinner, and my plate wasn't empty, there were consequences. Oh, silly parents! To think you could motivate a six-year-old boy not to play with his food. Can you stop the tides from rising? No! Can you stop the sun from setting? No! Well attempting to hasten my eating pace was on par with these.

Then one day, some brilliant TV network executive decided to broadcast the critically acclaimed series known as *Batman*. Now we all know that this version of Batman starring Adam West is not only the best version of Batman ever created, but is probably the best piece of dramatic enter-tainment ever produced on any medium ever. It was appointment television. At least for me (DVRs or even VCRs didn't exist). And that got my parents thinking. "What if we restricted the lad's access to *Batman* if he didn't clean his plate by the time the show aired?"

Yes, I know, you're all reading this and wishing you had a time machine so you could go back to 1966 and call Child Protective Services to haul my parents away (while you're at it, jump ahead to 1968 and make that TV executive put *Batman* back on the air). Unfortunately, you can't do that. And this is how I made the transition from someone who truly enjoyed his food (although not necessarily in the intended fashion) to someone who wolfed it down. It didn't matter whether I was hungry or full. No one ever had to wash my dishes again because the food would be gone before it hit the plate.

That was the turning point when I went from mind-FUL to mind-LESS eater. Not coincidentally, I also became a chubby kid. Many people have had similar experiences when the pleasures of eating were grabbed from them. Some people were coaxed to eat because there were starving

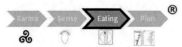

people in <insert-name-of-distant-land-to-which-you-couldn't-send-your-food>. Others were part of a family in which the TV blared constantly, even at meal time. And, you probably know people who had to gobble down some McNuggets while being shuttled between piano lessons and soccer practice (which I believe is American for football practice).

Regardless of how it happened, ever since the end of World War II, the balance of supply and demand for calories continuously shifted to encourage consumption of low quality calories as frequently and as quickly as possible.

With one simple change in our relationship with our food we can turn the tide back in our favor. That change is....wait for it...you've heard it before.

Eat Slowly and Stop Before You're Full

Well maybe it's actually two not-so-simple changes instead of one simple change, but I'm, going to make it easy for you. I'm going to simplify the concept and help you thoroughly enjoy your meal. The goal is to make you aware of the many cues associated with hunger. Furthermore, you should stop eating when you're at the point of satisfaction and well before the point of feeling full. If you're not already eating this way, this change should reduce the number of calories you eat.

I could wax poetic about the complex interplay of organs, muscles, neurotransmitters, enzymes, and hormones that are involved in the act of digestion. But first I'd need to figure out what the expression "wax poetic" actually means. These are two words that seem to have no business appearing adjacent to each other. Besides, the only poetic form I ever mastered was the limerick:

There once was a hormone named Cholecystokinin*
That's secreted in the small intestine.
It stimulates bile
And stops hunger for a while.
Without it rotundity's predestined.

Maybe "mastered" is too strong a word.

Instead, I'll "wax prosaic" and just say that when it comes to the feelings of satiety or fullness, it takes about twenty minutes for the symphony of signals to reach your brain and declare Surrender. This geezer-like pace plots against us and leads many of us to eat more food than we need or want. See this article for research confirming this statement minus the geezer reference.[62] Meanwhile, here's that prose I threatened.

Holy Slo Mo, Batman!

You're walking through your neighborhood and some car speeds down the street unreasonably fast. For geezers and other safety-minded individuals, the natural inclination may be to yell, "Slow Down!" How well do you think that will work? Even with the benefit of speed limits, people drive at the rate they've become accustomed to. Most people react the same way if you advise them to slow their eating pace (i.e., not at all). It's not that they don't want to; it's that they need more information. There are no speed limits for eating. However, there are some decent guidelines and an infinite number of strategies you can use to slow your pace, and I list many of them here. As a warning, one strategy contains such a long description, I documented it in the appendix of this book.

Before getting into any of the strategies, keep these two things in mind:

---

* a hormone that is secreted by cells in the duodenum and stimulates the release of bile into the intestine and the secretion of enzymes by the pancreas.

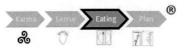

1. In the description of the Sense component, the plan introduces the pre-meal ritual that improves your mindset, rewires your brain, and reminds you to adjust to the new slow-eating habit.

2. Our target should be a minimum of fifteen to twenty minutes for a meal to allow that satiety mechanism to kick in. Stretch it out to thirty minutes or longer and you're an Abe Hellman-like pro.

With these as givens, here are strategies for slowing your pace:

1. Eat with your non-dominant hand.
2. Put your utensils and food down between bites.
3. Take smaller bites.
4. Drink more water during the meal.
5. Chew your food extensively. Count the number of times you usually chew your food before swallowing and extend that number by 10-25%
6. Dish out your normal meal size onto a smaller plate than usual. Set a timer for twenty minutes. No matter how long it takes you to complete the food you dished out, do not take seconds until the twenty minutes is up. Assess your hunger and only take more food if you're still hungry. Do not evaluate whether you are full or not. Instead, decide if you are hungry. This is my least favorite strategy. It focuses on the *before you're full* part at the expense of *eat slowly*. But if it works for you, by all means proceed.
7. Eat "Viking Style." When eating "Viking Style," don't use utensils. Just use your hands or dig in face first. Also, no napkins. Instead, wipe your face on the shoulder of the systkin (which I believe is Old Norse for sibling) next to you. But please, don't try this with hot soup or at a public restaurant. College dining halls are OK, though. At least that's what I am told.
8. Use chopsticks.
9. Be a truly mindful eater. This process allows you to regain the child-like wonder you once had about food, as if the experience

of eating was brand new, without the whole strained-peas-in-ear issue. In a nutshell, we're going to break down your meal (Break It Down!) so that you appreciate it as both the composed dish you are eating as well as the individual parts that make it up. You'll also focus on how your individual senses perceive the meal. Finally, you'll monitor how you feel while you eat. If this intrigues you, be sure to check out the full description in the Appendix. The mindful eating exercise is not something you need to do every time you eat. It is a good thing to do at several different meal settings (e.g., time of day, location, etc.).

These are some quick ideas on how to eat slowly. With your pace slowed down, the Boy Wonder has a declaration.

Holy Contentment, Batman!

Content, satisfied, fulfilled, sated. These are the sensations that we're aiming for. When you feel any of these, *The Karma Sense Eating Plan* asks that you stop. Do not pass Go! Do not collect another bite in your mouth. This is perhaps the plan's most challenging part. It's very difficult to know when we've reached this state. We have years of cultural and other pressures telling us to clean our plate, to have another helping. Not to do so is a waste. It's an insult to the people who prepared our food. Meanwhile it's well known, and research supported,[63] that portion sizes have grown over the years. These aren't easy tides to fight.

The "before you're full" feeling is also very hard to detect. It's so subjective. All of these different physiological processes that revolve around digestion take a while to kick in. It requires a keen connection between your brain and your body. It depends on all five of your senses as well as your common sense. It depends on your Karma Sense.

How do we deal with this? Mostly through trial and error. First, we need to reestablish the feeling that signals when it's time to stop eating. Strive for the point when you're no longer hungry. A good way to gauge

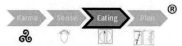

this is to take stock of how hungry you felt prior to eating. A better way is to follow the mindful eating exercise that you can still find in the Appendix (it hasn't moved).

When you've finished your first serving or it's been fifteen to twenty minutes since you started eating (whichever comes first), take stock of how you feel. Wait a few minutes. Do you feel the same? More content? Hungrier? Respond accordingly, deliberately, and slowly. What we're ultimately trying to achieve is the ability to counterattack all that cultural and marketing pressure to consume more calories. I know, consuming calories is pleasurable. But the feeling of contentment? That's getting it just right.

Whatever you ultimately do, eat more or quit, don't fret about whether or not you ate too much. Instead use the time following the meal to gauge how you feel every hour afterwards. Again, do you feel the same? More content? Stuffed? Hungry? If you get to five or six hours and you're still not hungry, you *may* have eaten too much in the previous meal. Or, you may just happen to have a small appetite.

I can't say it enough. This is a hard concept to master. The benefit, especially if you're trying to lose weight, is that if you do master it, you should lose weight without having to measure calories and macronutrients and without eliminating foods you love. The plan has other mantras to help you make further progress. But this one is a superhero.

Special Considerations

As we navigate through the Eating mantras, we'll look at how the mantras apply when trying to achieve some common goals. This subsection gives summary information if you're trying to lose weight, maintain your weight but eat healthier, or gain weight in the form of muscle.

Lose Weight

Implement this mantra as is. If you can master it, this mantra moves you towards your goal with no other dietary restrictions. If you want to lose faster or have difficulty losing, *The Karma Sense Eating Plan* should be implemented with further guidelines. A Health or Nutrition Coach ☺ can help you with this.

Maintain Weight but Eat Healthier

Implement this mantra as is, but monitor your weight. This mantra should not cause you to gain, but may cause you to lose weight. If you're moving too far in that direction, try increasing your portion size. Although eating faster will help, it's better to continue eating slowly. The advantages to digestion, sleep, and so on are just too good to give up.

Gain Weight in the Form of Muscle

Surprisingly, this mantra can be a good fit depending on your body fat percentage. However, if you're losing weight and not gaining muscle, you need to eat more.[*] If you're finding it hard to eat more, then eating faster may actually be a solution. By the way, if this is your problem, most people hate you. But not people who follow *The Karma Sense Eating Plan*. We have no room for hatin'.

Key Points

1. History, physiology, and the big food industry work together to encourage us to consume as many calories as we can as quickly as possible. The way to reverse this trend is to follow the mantra *Eat Slowly and Stop Before You're Full*.
2. One can adopt many strategies to *Eat Slowly*. The mindful approach is my favorite because it gives permission to reacquaint you with the joys of eating.

---

[*] You also may need more exercise.

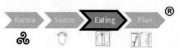

3. It takes some trial and error to *Stop Eating Before You're Full.* It is the most flexible way to reduce calorie intake and lose weight.

4. The mantra *Eat Slowly and Stop Before You're Full* makes sense for most people regardless of their nutrition, fitness, and health goals. People who want to gain weight in the form of muscle may need to modify this mantra.

Karma Sense in the Wild

My Cousin Arlene is a cool person. And I say this not solely because she is an early supporter of *The Karma Sense Eating Plan*. Everything Arlene does is cool. She's an artist (www.arelenew.com) who shares her skill by teaching her craft to adults in Southern California. She travels the US to deliver workshops on colored pencil techniques. She lives in one of America's hippest neighborhoods. As I said, cool.

Arlene's been a vegetarian for as long as I can remember, but isn't strident about it. She used to say that she only eats animals that don't have faces (e.g., clams and oysters which also happen to be the most sustainable and humane source of animal protein available). A while back she decided to drop mollusks from her diet too. The only animal products she eats now are eggs and food made from sheep or goat milk. Still no faces though.

Arlene ends every email with the salutation "Take care and breathe." I sometimes ask her stupid questions about that such as "Are we supposed to do them simultaneously or should we take care and then breathe?" She's kind enough to tolerate my teasing (at least she thinks it's teasing). But I have to admit, "Take care and breathe" is a succinct way of describing what I ask you to do in the chapter on the Sense component.

One side effect of Arlene reading about the plan is that it served as a motivator to improving her diet and increasing her activity. This isn't surprising. People often become inspired to adopt positive habits after they've been primed by new information on the subject.[64] It's sticking to these habits that can be the challenge.

One habit she jumped on quickly was mantra #1, *Eat Slowly and Stop Eating Before You're Full*. For her, the trick was to be sure to fully chew and swallow her food before putting more food in her mouth. In the past, she found that she would reload before swallowing the previous forkful. Eating that way is fairly common, especially when people feel rushed. But it can become a habit.

She also made other changes to her lifestyle but they were subtle, and

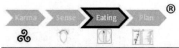

she said that even the people closest to her could not tell that she was doing anything different. Within six weeks, she lost an entire inch from her waistline. An inch in six weeks is significant progress. Cardiovascular disease is highly correlated with increased waist size.[65] Many physicians argue that waist size is the most important predictor of chronic disease, even more than weight or body mass index.

As stated, *Eat Slowly and Stop Eating Before You're Full* is not the only change Arlene made. It was significant enough for her to single it out. Regardless of whether it's responsible for her decreased waist-size, there's no doubt that it made her healthier.

We continue on to mantra #2 in the next chapter. Same Bat time. Same Bat channel.

Mantra #2: Eat Protein in Every Meal

Executive Summary

In this chapter, we move to the second of five mantras in the Eating component, Eat Protein in Every Meal. We'll talk about how much protein is right for you, various food options, some of the myths about protein consumption, and I'm sure some totally irrelevant stuff as well.

And speaking of irrelevant stuff.

Disclaimer

I am not a doctor nor do I play one on TV. In fact, I've been told I have a face for radio, the voice of an author, and the writing skills of those thousand monkeys they keep threatening to throw in a room full of typewriters. But the important thing to focus on here is the part that I am not a doctor.

Therefore, the information I pass to you throughout this book should not be considered a prescription for disease treatment or as medical advice. It is however based on sound research and common sense and as previously stated, I am trained and experienced in the fields of wellness and nutrition. Still, I highly recommend you consult your doctor before performing any radical changes to your diet. The good thing for most people is that *The Karma Sense Eating Plan* is far from nutritionally radical. But it might be considered radical in a Spicoli surfer-dude sort of way.

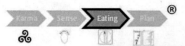

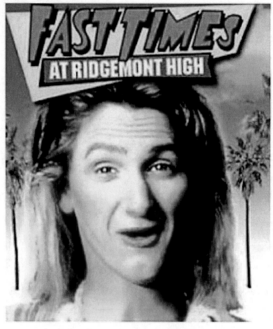

Figure 23 Radical[66,67]

Now, what follows actually does have some relevance to the topic of Eat Protein in Every Meal.

How I Became a Nutrition Wonk

When we left off discussing mantra #1, Eat Slowly and Stop Before You're Full, I flipped from scrappy rambunctious kid to chubby fella who shopped in the husky section. From that chapter, you know that this transition was tied to a Batman caper. I don't know which of Batman's supervillains to blame, but I went from being practically a male model

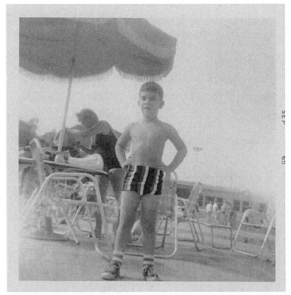

Figure 24 Practically a Male Model[68]

to someone who could have been The Penguin's stunt double.

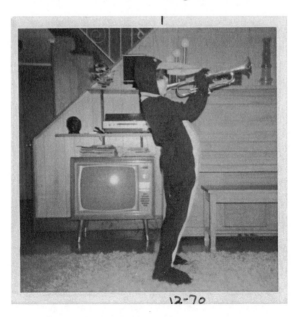

Figure 25 Holy Blow Hard, Batman![69]

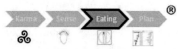

But seriously, the band uniform may mask it a little but I was definitely overweight. There were never any attempts by me or anyone else to change my corpulent trajectory. When I was nine years old, I started going to sleep-away camp during the summers. I always returned home thinner than when I left. This was mostly due to a combination of portion control (no second helpings) and less access to food in general (no fridge or pantry to explore). Oh yeah, and the food was kind of gross.

Here was mantra #1 in action; at least the Stop Eating Before Full part. Despite dropping those pounds, within a few months, my weight rebounded.

When I was thirteen, someone brought home a book on the Atkins Diet.[70] I wasn't the only one struggling with weight in my house, but I'm pretty sure I was the target audience for this new addition to our library. My parents knew that no book was safe from my eyes when it entered our home. This led to some awkward moments, but no need to go there. Anyway, I read the Atkins Diet book and I had an epiphany. A full description of the diet is beyond the scope of this book, but it was perfect for my "on the spectrum" brain because it was science-y (ketosis!) and rule-based, and therefore, easy to systemize (see my Origin Story early in this book). For the purposes of this discussion all you need to know is that it was a high protein, no-to-low carb diet that created great controversy because it was so counter to current nutritional dogma at the time. It also created results.

Within months, I went from fat, awkward, prepubescent nerd to skinny, awkward, pubescent nerd. Although the results are quick with the Atkins Diet, they are not sustainable. Your body needs carbohydrates (and excels at processing them if you follow mantra #3, Eat Whole Food Carbohydrates After Vigorous Exercise). Fortunately for me, raging hormones took over and fought back the tides of my return to hamburgers, french fries, ice cream and food I no longer wanted to play with. But two things kicked in:

1. My forever obsession with nutrition, physiology, and health.
2. My recognition of protein as a major source of my personal good nutrition and well-being.

And, as usual, I'll try to force fit this back story into the subject at hand.

Eat Protein in Every Meal

This mantra's detailed description has a fair amount of geekiness and complexity. If you're not interested in how the sausage (processed protein) is made, here's the bottom line.

If you're a woman, aim for one serving of protein per meal. If you're a man, aim for two servings per meal. A serving is about the size of your palm. Alternatively, aim for twenty to thirty grams per meal for women and forty to sixty grams for men. If your goal is to achieve the best health and body composition simultaneously, it's very hard to do without pumping up the protein. Furthermore, because protein is so filling, it's hard to eat more unless you spread it throughout the day. So, Eat Protein in Every Meal. It is perfectly safe for most people. You won't overdose on protein as long as you follow the other mantras. The only exception is if you have a kidney condition, in which case check with a doctor. Contrary to popular belief, no research has ever uncovered a connection between high protein consumption and kidney problems for people whose kidneys are healthy.

There are many subtleties you can obsess over to meet the Eat Protein in Every Meal mantra and I'll give you the opportunity to do so later in this chapter (e.g., what is a meal? does any protein count?). But if all you care about are the basics of mantra #2, you just read everything you need to know.

On to the Promised Geekfest

The Atkins Diet deserves criticism. In fact, even Dr. Atkins thought so. Over the years, he changed the basic principles of the diet towards a

---

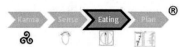

more mainstream (and healthful) balance of macronutrients. In the meantime, many versions of high protein—low-carb diet plans followed. These plans tend to work for the following reasons:

1. Initially, since you're not taking in carbs, you deplete the carbo-hydrates stored in your body in the form of glycogen. Water is a byproduct of the chemical reaction required to do this. The depletion of carbohydrates causes an initial rapid weight loss as your body gets rid of all the water that helped to store glycogen. People who carry their weight in the middle start to lose some bloat (inches around the waist) as well.

2. The moment of truth begins. Once you're out of glycogen, your body starts burning other sources of energy, usually fat. Many people start to feel sluggish as the body transitions to this new energy source, and this is when they quit. Others are so inspired by initial weight loss that they stick it out.

3. For those who stick it out, the carb cravings die down. The weight loss continues but at a slower rate. The simple equation of weight loss kicks in; calories consumed are less than calories burned.

High protein—low-carb diets are elimination diets. Focusing on protein is especially successful for elimination diets because protein fills you up and is slow to digest. But overall, diet plans that remove entire food groups tend to bring on weight loss because limited variety usually means lower calorie consumption. This weight loss is not absolute, as certain lifestyles allow enough calorie-dense foods to elevate calorie intake. But this food-group-restriction attribute is the reason there are so many specialty diets that support weight loss. Paleo diets. Gluten-free diets. Even the Cookie Diet. You can lose weight on all of them. But most of the weight loss is due to the simple equation (calorie intake is less than calorie expenditure).

In fact, as I said earlier, the concept of *The Karma Sense Eating Plan* jolted me awake in the middle of the night. Another brilliant idea that once came to me this way was the "Mad Lib Diet" (What? Am I the only one who dreams about diet plans?).

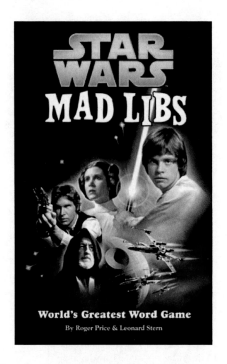

Figure 26 The Star Wars Version Only Allows Foods You Can Order From the Mos Eisley Cantina[71]

The Mad Lib Diet worked like this. Each page is linked to one week of the diet. The page prompted you to write down things like "name of vegetable" or "third favorite junk food" or even just "verb" for physical activity. When you filled in all the blanks, you could read it back and get your eating instructions for the week. Page one was associated with week one. Page two with week two and so on. There's a good chance that some people would lose weight because of the food elimination theory. And, like any good diet guru, I'd exploit the people who were successful and ignore the people who were not for the sake of selling more Mad Lib pads. Fortunately, this was not one of the ideas that stuck the next morning. (Note to Penguin Group USA, LLC: contact me at daveyh@livelongleadlong.com if interested.) (Note to Reader: Penguin

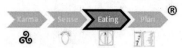

Group USA, LLC is the publisher of Mad Libs and is not affiliated with the Batman supervillain or the dapper fellow depicted in the photo earlier in this chapter.)

MAD LIBS ☺ Diet

BREAKFAST

Week 1

_____ minutes after you wake up, do _____ _____. Then make an
(Number)   **(Number) (Exercise)**

omelet using three _____ eggs and chopped _____. You may also
                          (Animal)   **(Vegetable)**

have unlimited cups of _____. If at the end of breakfast you feel _____,
                          (Hot Beverage)   **(Emotion)**

you may also have a _____ piece of _____ as long as you follow it up with
                          (Size)   **(Food)**

some _____ within _____ _____ of eating.
      (Verb ending in –ing)   **(Number) (Units of Time)**

Figure 27 Sample Page From the Mad Lib Diet[72]

Tell Me More About the Amount of Protein I Should Eat

Now I'm going to tell you *exactly* how much protein to eat—except for the "exactly" part. In compliance with the *Keep America's Nutrition Experts Gainfully Employed Act of 2012*, there is no clear-cut answer. But I'll drill down for you.

First you have the recommended daily amount from a variety of official channels such as the U.S government (e.g., Centers for Disease Control)[73]:

- Babies need about ten grams a day.
- School-age kids need nineteen to thirty-four grams a day.
- Teenage boys need up to fifty-two grams a day.
- Teenage girls need forty-six grams a day.
- Adult men need about fifty-six grams a day.
- Adult women need about forty-six grams a day.

These equate to a target of 0.8 grams of protein per kilogram of body weight or 0.36 grams per pound. Then there are the special cases such as:

- Pregnant or Breastfeeding- seventy-one grams a day.
- Athlete - add 50% more a day.
- Dieting - varies but around 30-35% of calories from protein.
- Vegan/Vegetarian - no difference, but be mindful that you eat enough. Of particular concern is that many plant-based sources of protein do not digest as easily as animal sources. Therefore, some nutrition experts recommend an increase of 20-35% over the above recommendations (e.g., fifty-four to sixty-two grams for an adult woman).

No one as yet has offered protein recommendations for Infant Vegetarian Athletes.

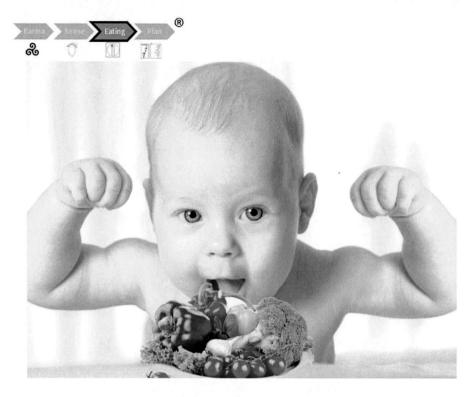

Figure 28 Oh, they exist. They exist!!![74]

With *The Karma Sense Eating Plan*, we're aiming for 0.75 grams to 1.25 grams per pound of body weight (1.7 to 3.3 grams per kilogram of body weight). This target also answers the question of what constitutes a meal. If you're goal is 120 grams of protein a day and you get thirty grams in each of three meals, you'll need a snack meal or two to get you to your goal. Yes, this is decidedly more protein than government agency recommendations. The difference is due to two reasons; politics and ignorance. The politics, which are tremendously complex, add too much bad karma to this good karma zone, so I'm choosing to ignore it for now. If you're interested in my view, I bloviate on the subject incessantly in multiple blog posts about the Healthcare Industrial Complex.[75] The ignorance, which exists on both sides of the argument, is explored soon. First we'll discuss protein sources.

Where Should I Get All This Protein Goodness?

As noted in this book more times than you can shake a stick at (which isn't really a very useful activity if you ask me), *The Karma Sense Eating Plan* is designed to be inclusive. Its aim is to allow you to eat the foods you enjoy most. That being said, if your Karma Sense goal is to gain better health while creating a better world, here are some basic guidelines on optimal protein sources:

- The less processed the better. If your protein comes in a package that includes an ingredient list, it's processed. The more ingredients on that list, the more processed it is. If you want to eat processed food, aim for foods with ingredients you can pronounce. Processed proteins such as cold cuts, hot dogs, and Slim Jims are bad for the planet and bad for your health. I realize that last statement is a gross generalization and throughout this book I sincerely avoid gross generalizations. In the case of processed protein I feel justified. I choose to generalize in response to an equally gross and incorrect generalization that, because processed proteins are bad for you, all proteins are bad.
- The more humane and sustainable, the better. For some people, the heartburn they avoid by eating protein from animals that are well-treated is cancelled out by the heartburn they get from the price of labels saying things such as "pasture-raised" or "grass-fed." It's a valid point. Fortunately, sustainable options are finding their way onto shelves of discount grocers and warehouse clubs. The more we buy, the cheaper they'll become.

Here are some more specific suggestions with notes:

Protein	Note
Lean Meat	Beef, Chicken, Turkey, Pork, Bison, Venison. Grass and pasture fed preferred (to be discussed with mantra #5)
Fish/Seafood	Wild caught from low in the food chain preferred

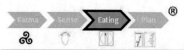

Protein	Note
	Cold water fish help with mantra #5.
Eggs	Laid from cage-free chickens with natural diet preferred
Dairy	Greek yogurt, Cheese. High-fat content can be an issue if weight loss is a goal
Plant Sources	Beans, Lentils, Peas, Nuts, Seeds, Quinoa, Soy, Buckwheat, Quorn, Seitan
Crickets/Insects and other Creepy Crawlies	Sustainable and nutrient-dense, while being inexpensive and low in calories. **Gross out your friends.**

Table 4 Protein Options

Note that if your goals are more than simply achieving better health (e.g., losing weight) you may need more guidance on optimal protein choices. I'll cover how to deal with specific and technical goals when I introduce the Plan component. But let's move on.

Addressing Myths About Protein

There are so many myths about how excessive protein affects your health. Let's bust those myths right now.

...Too Much Protein is Bad for Your Kidneys

Busted. In 1983 scientists discovered that the more protein you consume, the higher your glomerular filtration rate (GFR) which is a key function of your kidneys. Based on this, they assumed that increased protein stresses kidneys. However, hundreds of follow-up studies (including this one) show no link to increased GFR and problems with healthy kidneys due to protein consumption.[76] These tests used amounts higher than the maximum range of 1.25 grams per pound of body weight that I'm suggesting. I repeat, if you have kidney problems, consult your doctor before changing your protein intake. Healthy kidneys? OK.

...Too Much Protein is Bad for Osteoporosis

Busted. Protein increases your body's acidity and it was hypothesized that the increased acidity leached calcium from your bones. However, multiple studies show the opposite is true.[77] Diets rich in protein actually improve calcium absorption and prevent or delay the effects of osteoporosis. Furthermore, if you follow mantra #3, you'll neutralize the effects of excess acidity in the body.

...High Protein Diets Have a Positive Effect in Managing Blood Glucose of Type 2 Diabetics

Confirmed. Numerous studies show high protein diets help fight obesity and Type 2 Diabetes. Here's an example.[78]

...High Protein Diets are Bad for the Heart. Low-Fat Diets are Superior.

Busted. A Scientific American article I reference in the book's Notes, accompanying rebuttal by Dr. Dean Ornish, re-rebuttal by the author do a great job demonstrating how contentious this issue is. The whole sad tale is at the same link. But while the children argue over minor details, let's focus on where they agree. High-quality protein is good for you. The evidence that high protein diets are bad for you is weak.[79]

...Eating More Protein Causes Cancer

Inconclusive. The research is convoluted. The source of protein certainly matters. Processed meat, for example seems to increase the likelihood of cancer. Plant sources seem to decrease the likelihood. Unless, of course, that plant source is soy which is linked to cancer when eaten in certain quantities. Except for those cases where soy is a shown to prevent cancer. See what I mean by convoluted? It's a case in which the research doesn't clarify much of anything.

I recommend that you do your best to understand your personal risk for certain types of cancer and explore the issue with your doctor (see

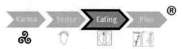

previous disclaimer) and a nutrition expert (such as yours truly). This _article_ by Examine.com does a good job of explaining the issue.[80] It is very detailed, but at least Examine is a source of reason.

...You Definitely Lose Weight with a High Protein Diet

Busted. High protein diets tend to work because they assume a reduction in carbohydrate consumption. Protein is satiating and when carbs are managed, calorie intake tends to decrease. If you still include carbs as a major part of your diet, weight loss is less than assured. This is especially true if you opt for fattier proteins. So that thick crust meat-lovers pizza is not your best option. Mantra #4, Eat Whole Food Carbohydrates After Vigorous Exercise includes a strategy on how to manage carb intake for people interested in losing and maintaining their weight.

...High Protein−Low-Carb Improves Insulin Sensitivity (Which is a Good Thing)

Busted, although mostly true. Insulin sensitivity improves because there is less glucose for insulin to respond to and because of likely weight loss. But if you go too extreme with your high protein−low-carb imple-mentation, the body will switch to an insulin resistance mode.[81] This is a protective mechanism which ensures that any available glucose finding its way through your body is available to your brain.

...With Plant-Based Proteins You Must Consume Complementary Pro-teins Together In Order To Get Full Benefit

Busted. It is correct that many plant sources do not have the full profile of amino acids that make up a complete protein. This is why vegans often consume combinations like beans-and-rice or peanut butter on toast. However, the American Dietetic Association and similar organizations internationally now take the _position_ that you're okay as long as you eat the complete profile some time throughout the day.[82]

Busted. *The Karma Sense Eating Plan* can coexist with high protein lifestyles. At this point you know that Karma Sense has an inclusive mindset and does not exclude specific foods. The plan encourages higher intake of protein than the minimum recommended by government agencies, but its target is well within the range advocated by many nutrition experts. Furthermore, *The Karma Sense Eating Plan* suggests control of carbohydrate intake for those who want to lose weight, but recognizes that carbohydrates have an important role for overall health.

Special Considerations

As with mantra #1, Eat Slowly and Stop Before Full, this section explores how people with different goals adjust the mantra of Eat Protein in Every Meal.

Lose Weight

Implement this mantra as is.

Maintain Weight but Eat Healthier

Implement this mantra as is.

Gain Weight in the Form of Muscle

Implement this mantra as is. You may need to aim towards the higher target of 1.25 grams per pound of body weight.

Key Points

1. If you're a woman, aim for one serving of protein per meal. If you're a man, aim for two servings per meal. A serving is about the size of your palm. Alternatively, aim for twenty to thirty grams per meal for women and forty to sixty grams for men.

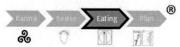

2. Target daily consumption is 0.75 grams to 1.25 grams of protein per pound of body weight.

3. If you have kidney issues, consult with your physician before changing your protein intake.

4. Protein consumption at the plan's recommended level is safe and supports optimal health for people with healthy kidneys.

Karma Sense in the Wild

Sharon Lewis is a friend of mine and a fellow Integrative Health Coach who struggled with obesity for most of her life. For as long as she remembers, Sharon worked very hard to manage her weight with a combination of exercise and diet, but had little success. Metabolic syndrome and other related issues worked against her efforts to raise her metabolism and shed weight. In addition, as a "lean in" level executive in the high tech field, her stress levels were through the roof.

With all other options exhausted and a continued vision of a healthier self, Sharon elected bariatric surgery, a procedure in which the digestive system is physically manipulated to stimulate weight loss. Specifically, she chose a procedure called the gastric sleeve, in which part of the stomach is removed. This was a commitment to a severe calorie restricted diet, but calorie restriction alone would not lead to triumph. To succeed, she needed to include a regimen of exercise, mindfulness, and support group participation.

Bariatric surgery is not trivial. It's usually pursued after all other options are exhausted. It is considered major surgery and can have many complications. According to one meta-analysis, the success rate of bariatric surgery is difficult to track.[83] But individual studies report success rates as high as 93% in morbidly obese patients and 57% in the super-obese.[84] Even for the morbidly obese, these results are not optimal when you consider the potential risks of major surgery.

Sharon is one of the success stories. She is able to channel the dedication she always devoted to her career to the process of becoming healthy. What does any of this have to do with Eat Protein in Every Meal?

People who elect bariatric surgery have to micromanage macronutrients and micronutrients (say that five times fast). There is no room for error in meal size, frequency, and composition. When Sharon kindly agreed to tolerate my curiosity on the subject, she emphasized the importance of protein whenever she eats. She knows that carbohydrates and fats are important, but protein deficiency can have the most deleterious effects. These include, but are not limited to,

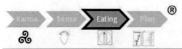
muscle loss, hormonal imbalance, damage to hair, skin, and nails, anemia, sleep loss, headache, and so on. It is a list so long and scary, it begins to sound like one of those pharmaceutical ads. One advantage of the gastric sleeve over other procedures is that the sleeve promotes normal absorption of vitamins and minerals. This ensures that protein is properly digested and processed. It also means Sharon can fill out her nutritional needs with high quality supplements.

That's what this story has to do with mantra #2. Even when your ability to eat is highly restricted, Eat Protein in Every Meal. And if you'd like to hear more about Sharon's story or take advantage of her wisdom in becoming healthier against all odds, contact her and visit her website at www.weightothink.com.

Mantra #3: Eat More Vegetables and Fruits

Executive Summary

In this chapter, we move to the third of five mantras in the Eating component. You may recall that *The Karma Sense Eating Plan* is designed to make you happy, healthy and oh yeah, save the world. While the other four mantras and the Sense component target your happiness and health, and the Karma component focuses on saving the world, mantra #3, Eat More Vegetables and Fruits, supports all of these goals. We'll talk about the reason I make this claim, how much of this goodness to strive for, why I say "vegetables and fruits" instead of the more common "fruits and vegetables," and ideas to help you if you think vegetables are nasty.

I'll also explain why you probably think they're nasty. You'll be happy to know this chapter won't talk much about fictional superheroes. However, it does discuss a real life superhero.

Your Mother

NOTE: Despite the low-brow content you've come to expect in The Karma Sense Eating Plan, "Your mother" jokes will not be employed in this discussion. Even I have standards. Knock-knock jokes are still on the table, however.

I'm sure your mother is super in many ways. She also is a hero. But a superhero is more than the sum of these two parts and when it comes to forming your sense of taste, your mom fits the bill.

Now, for the sake of establishing the scope of this discussion, by "taste" I specifically mean the act of tasting things you put in your mouth and not aesthetic taste. Because, when it comes to how a mom can affect your aesthetic taste, it can be a real train wreck.

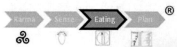

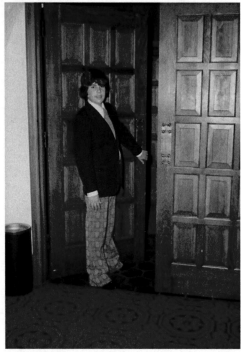

Figure 29 Pants Selected by Mom. Size "Husky".[85]

Who wouldn't think they were in for a good time passing through THAT door?

In the genre of superheroes, your mom is like Professor X. If you're mature, you may be wondering who Professor X is (and if you're mature I'm wondering why you're still reading this but thank you for doing so.) Professor X can read minds (just like Mom!). But his greatest strength is his role as mentor for the X-Men. Professor X has little control but significant influence over those rapscallions. Your mom has little control over your sense of taste, but she has significant influence. Here's how it plays out:

- When you were conceived, specific genes determined how you would perceive taste. Take cilantro for example. People love it or hate it. And <u>research</u> shows that your opinion is tied directly to a specific gene variation.[86] Another example is that of the "supertaster" (as opposed to normal tasters). Supertasters perceive undesirable qualities in a broad range of food from gin to grapefruit to green tea. But this ability is not just limited to foods that start with the letter "g." Alas, poor supertasters, coffee, India Pale Ales and several other foods are also on their yuck list.[87] Although supertasting is linked to genetics, it occurs more often with women. A child's sex is determined by the dad, so mom shouldn't take all the blame for this one. As an aside, if I had the choice to heighten one of my five senses for a superpower, I think the sense of taste might be the lamest. "Hmmm, tastes like rotten fish...Must be The Penguin!"

- During gestation, fetal nutrition is mostly passed from Mom's blood to the developing baby's blood. The sense of taste is not stimulated. But, according to one study, the fetus has a tendency to swallow amniotic fluid.[88] Since amniotic fluid takes on the flavor of the mother's diet, this exposure impacts how we later perceive taste.

- After a baby is born, Mom has more opportunity as breast milk picks up the flavors of the mother's diet. If the mom chooses to feed with formula, she delegates the flavor responsibility to a multinational corporation, usually Abbott, Mead Johnson, or Nestle. (NOTE: There is nothing wrong with delegating the flavor responsibility to a multinational corporation. It's your choice. As adults, we do it to ourselves all the time. My modest proposal is that until your children are able to make their own food choices, taste test anything you did not make yourself, including baby formula. Babies of the world, I'm on your side.)

- The final opportunity for influencing taste happens when we develop our own free will. (Usually) Mom wants us to eat certain foods because they're good for us. We push back because we think these foods taste like our gym socks. And your mom didn't have my Live Long Lead Long series of posts about "Readiness to Change" available to her so she could be more successful in her

---

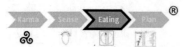

attempts.[89,90] We all know how this played out, but it's probably best depicted in this <u>scene</u> from the documentary series, *Leave it to Beaver*.

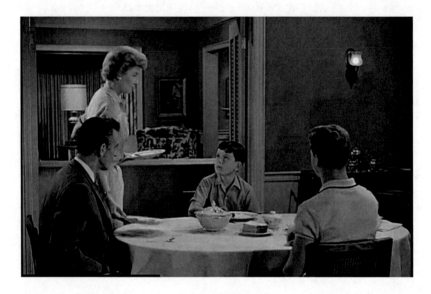

Figure 30 What Family Dinner Looked Like for Approximately 0.00001% of the U.S. Population.[91,92]

This is one of those times in which a printed description just can't live up to what actually happens. But if you don't watch the video referenced in the Endnotes, here are some of the tactics Theodore Cleaver used to avoid eating his Brussels sprouts:

- The stall – just wait Mom out.
- The fake sickness – distract Mom and aim for her sympathy.
- The spread – move the vegetables around the plate so it looks like there was some action.
- The hide – in this case, his shirt pocket.
- The complain – an exercise in futility.

What Theodore Cleaver and so many of us eventually learned is that Brussels sprouts and many vegetables are an acquired taste. There are a lot of valid reasons why people don't like to eat them. If you're one of these people, I spend time in this chapter explaining why and how you can change.

If you're already a convert, I'll get into the specifics of mantra #3 now so that you can read the rest of this chapter with a smug look on your face knowing how much cooler you are than vegetable haters (This is an attempt at peer pressure in case logic isn't working). So, without further ado, mantra #3...

Eat More Vegetables and Fruits

Your mission, which you should accept, is to eat seven to ten servings of vegetables and fruits per day. In general, eat more vegetables than fruits. When I discuss the Special Considerations to which you've become accustomed, I'll get more specific.

Vegetables are preferred because of their lower calorie density (calories per gram is low) relative to nutrient density (vitamins, minerals, fiber and phytonutrients per gram are high). It's best to spread this consumption throughout the day by including them in every meal. This is not a requirement, but try to eat enough by the end of the day. Unlike mantra #2, Eat Protein in Every Meal, this mantra carries the same serving size whether you're a man or woman. Here are guidelines on the meaning of "a serving:"

- One (1) cup green leafy vegetables
- One (1) medium-sized piece of fruit (the size of an adult fist)
- Half (½) cup chopped raw fruit, whole berries, or vegetables

When we discussed mantra #2, we dug into the controversy among experts about how much protein we should eat. Nutrition experts universally agree that we should eat more vegetables and fruits. If a controversy exists, it's what we know we should do versus what we want to do. We prefer other foods to vegetables. When we dish out food onto our plate, we don't leave much real estate for the vegetable to move in. When the plate is dished out for us, the vegetable is often what we

---

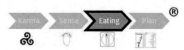

leave on the plate when we finish. I understand this preference. I know that, for the vegetable averse or even the vegetable ambivalent, building up to ten servings a day seems insurmountable. If you'll bear with me, we'll work through this later in the chapter.

First we need to talk about a unique and important characteristic of mantra #3. You're reading *The Karma Sense Eating Plan* because you want to be healthier, happier and, oh yeah, save the world (you're not reading it, I assume, because it is a great piece of modern literature). The plan achieves these three goals by linking good deeds and gratitude (Karma and Sense components) to eating behaviors (Eating component). Adopting the Eating behaviors improves your health and contributes to your happiness, but it's the plan's other aspects that help save the world. Only one of the five mantras in the Eating component works towards making you healthier, making you happier AND saving the world. This behavior is Eat More Vegetables and Fruits. In the following discussion, I defend this claim and I do so with some sweet Kung Fu moves that include research, common sense, facts, allegory, emotion, and Mom.

Eating More Vegetables and Fruits Makes You Healthy

Mom is right. Vegetables and fruits are good for you. Study after study demonstrates this. They fight disease (studies).[93] They manage your weight (study).[94] They make you look good (study).[95] It is known, Khaleesi. I will assert this no further.

<Kung Fu Swish sound effect>

Eating More Vegetables and Fruits Makes You Happy

I'll lean on my usual crutch, peer-reviewed research, to back this claim. While it's true that the salty-sweet-fatty sensation of bacon-and-ranch-flavored-chocolate-covered-cheese-puffs can give you a temporary boost in mood, the crash is usually just as fast. This causes sadness and increases your craving for salty-sweet-fatty foods. According to one study, consuming a minimum of seven servings of vegetables and fruits gives this same kick and lasts longer.[96] It's the time-released version of the junk food high.

There are several reasons why. First, many of the ingredients in unhealthy foods that enhance mood are also in vegetables and fruits. Second, vegetables and fruits contain other naturally occurring substances such as fiber, vitamins, minerals, and phytonutrients (also known as "other goodies") that regulate and slow down the absorption of these ingredients. Furthermore, the fiber, vitamins, minerals, and other goodies (also known as "phytonutrients") contain mood-enhancing properties of their own. Fiber leads to satiation. Folic acid, a B vitamin found in abundance in broccoli and other vegetables, has a direct link to positive moods, and its deficiency is directly correlated to depression (study).[97] Magnesium, a mineral found in dark green leafy vegetables like spinach, also prevents depression and anxiety (study!).[98] And, polyphenols, a family of phyto-goodies (also known as "other nutrients"), fight depression and Alzheimer's disease (guess what!).[99]

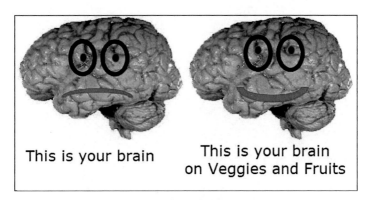

This is your brain   This is your brain
                            on Veggies and Fruits

Figure 31 fMRI Results of Two Brains Based on Diet. True Story.[100]

<Kung Fu *Swish-Swish* sound effect>

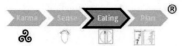

Eating More Vegetables and Fruits Saves the World

I evoked Mom to push us through the *health* claim. I leaned on research to carry us through the *happy* claim. To make my case that Eating More Vegetables and Fruits will help save the world, I'll depend on common sense, facts, allegory, and emotion. But first, housekeeping.

Housekeeping

For this discussion, the point I assert is that plant sources of nutrition (e.g., veggies, fruits, grains, legumes, nuts) are better than animal sources for the environment and other living creatures. I make no value judgment as to whether meat consumption is good or bad. I do, however, encourage you to eat more vegetables and fruit in exchange for, and at the expense of, animal-based nutrition.

One reason *The Karma Sense Eating Plan* guides you in this direction is because it's a better choice for you, your loved ones, the population at large, other sentient beings, and the planet. Sound familiar? How about now?

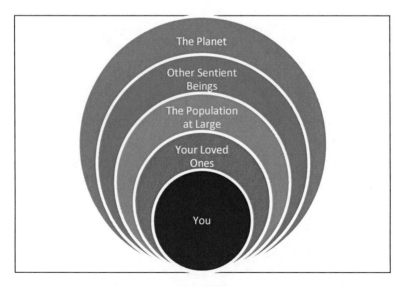

Figure 32 Yikes! Not the "Save the World" Model Again!

People have different priorities when it comes to saving the world and we'll explore these in the hopes that some combination will match your world-saving view. We'll use the Save the World Model as we move along.

Also keep in mind that while the world of plant-based food is not limited to vegetables and fruits, the more carb-olicious and fat-tastic sources (i.e. grains and nuts respectively) are discussed as part of mantras #4 and #5 as well as other random places in this book because sometimes I simply couldn't keep them under control. They're mischievous in that way.

Okay, now we can discuss why plants are better for you.

You

See Healthy and Happy above. If you are the center of your world and you are happy and healthy, the "save the world" part is done.

Your Loved Ones

I'm in the mood for a table. Aren't you?

Which Situation Is Best For Your Loved Ones?			
Are You		Happy?	
		Yes	No
Healthy?	Yes		
	No		

Table 5 Green (or Solid) Means Good. Red (or Hatched) Means Bad.

The Population At Large

It would be great at this point if there was some research I could reference demonstrating that happy and healthy populations are better global citizens. There isn't. But isn't it just common sense? Let's explore the Happy-Healthy theme a little bit anyway.

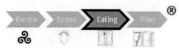

Relying on research to demonstrate that happiness helps save the world is a losing battle. Not because the research contradicts the claim but because the research is a mess. The definition of happiness is too subjective. Research sponsors use the definition that best suits their specific purposes. Socialists measure it their way. Libertarians measure it their way. Moderates measure it both ways and average it out.

For this discussion, I define happiness the same way Supreme Court Justice Potter Stewart defined hard-core pornography, "I know it when I see it."[101] Another thing I know is that individual happiness breeds more happiness. If you're happy, the people around you get happier and so on. By the time you move six degrees away, even Kevin Bacon is happy. That's good for the population at large.

Meanwhile, as it relates to health, there are all sorts of quirky studies. While they may disagree on measures, methods and next steps, they all agree that healthy populations live longer (duh), are more productive, create less global instability, consume more and, therefore improve the economy. No one is rooting to lead the world in chronic disease.

I hope we can just agree that a happy and healthy population stands a better chance of saving the world than a bunch of disease-ridden grumpy-pants.

Other Sentient Beings

You don't have to be a vegetarian to believe that animals would be better off if we ate less of them. Some attempt to undermine this position, but they usually use specious logic. If you can't think of any of the lame arguments they'd use, good for you. You're pure of soul.

Which leaves the Planet.

The Planet

I could focus solely on the issue of global warming and climate change to make this point. But everyone already knows that:

"So-called 'global warming' is just a secret ploy by wacko tree-huggers to make America energy independent, clean our air and water, improve the fuel efficiency of our vehicles, kick-start 21st-century industries, and make our cities safer and more livable. Don't let them get away with it!" – Chip Giller Founder of Grist.org,[102]

But seriously, it's irrelevant to this conversation whether climate and atmosphere changes are forces of nature or forces of knuckleheads.

I'll explain why by telling you about my son and his very own superpower. When he was very young, he could debate with people of any age, use logic and facts to convince them he was right, and then as soon as they came to his side, he'd switch. He'd take the other side. He'd reassemble the facts and logic that his "opponent" used and shake their confidence in their thought process. This quote best represents this skill:

"The test of a first-rate intelligence* is the ability to hold two opposed ideas in mind at the same time and still retain the ability to function." - F. Scott Fitzgerald[103]

The same technique can easily apply to the debate about which type of food is more sustainable. Don't believe me? Try me! I've been trained by the best.

In the end, it's a discussion of values. And a debate over values is as close to a religious debate as you can get without it actually being a religious debate. Sometimes it is one and the same. Has a religious

---

*It is true that I am implying that both my sons have a first rate intelligence by invoking this quote. Like their sense of taste, it is a quality they get from their mom.

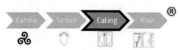

debate ever concluded with a nice clean resolution other than the occasional agree-to-disagree?

How Eating More Plants Saves the World Even If You Don't Believe in Global Warming

Here are the irrefutable facts. Plants are lower on the food chain. The lower on the food chain, the less energy and fewer resources are consumed. Plants can grow closer to the consumer, and this also conserves energy. I can grow spinach in my backyard. My city neighbors might have problems if I raised cows. In general, plants require much less processing and packaging than animals. The carrots and bananas that pass through my door look pretty much like they did in their natural setting. The chicken usually is separated from its feathers, head, and feet by the time it arrives home. It's wrapped in cellophane and other petroleum based products that never decay. Finally, plants pollute less than animals, whether it's gas in the air or waste on the ground. Animals have a bigger (literal and figurative) footprint.

How Eating More Plants Saves the World If You Do Believe in Global Warming

For people who DO believe greenhouse gasses exist, the following chart (Figure 33 Plants - Good for Everyone.) by the Environmental Working Group illustrates how eating more plants is better for the planet.

A picture is worth a 1,000 words, unless you're my son. He'll remind you that while the chart is accurate, it's misleading. You have to eat a lot of broccoli to get the same amount of energy you get from a slice of ham. If you were on a deserted island with one food and the choice was broccoli or ham, you'd survive a lot longer with the cured meat. In fact, if you substitute the ham with Ben & Jerry's Chubby Hubby ice cream, you'd still live longer than with broccoli. (Note to Self: Remember to volunteer for the desert island Chubby Hubby experiment).

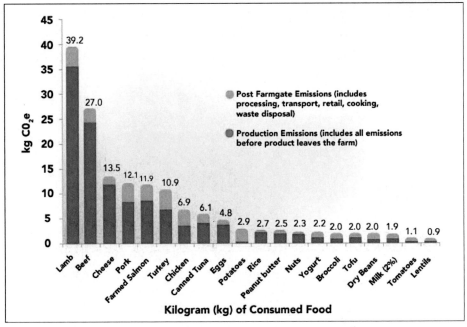

Figure 33 Plants - Good for Everyone[104].

So, the table is misleading. If you sort the data by calorie density, pork, chicken, and fish start to mingle among the plant-based foods in emission output. Lamb and beef are still way far to the left (leftist sheep! They probably believe in global warming).

The table is also misleading because it doesn't consider invasive and destructive species in the wild such as deer, wild boar, and snakeheads. Leaving these populations to their own devices causes more damage to the environment than killing them in moderation. Once dead, it would be more tragic to let them go to waste.

This conflicting information makes my head spin. Now you see what it was like living with that kid.

In the end, we learn that data like this tries to convert the intangible, intertwined force of all living things (←blatant Star Wars reference) into discrete pieces of information. That's not how real life works (much to

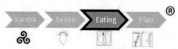

my chagrin—see my Origin Story). So we have to depend on common sense in cases where data alone can't serve. But if using facts, logic, and common sense doesn't convince you that to Eat More Vegetables and Fruits makes you healthy, happy, and, oh yeah, saves the world, then at least listen to your mom. She only wants what's best and, just like Professor X, she believes you *can* save the world.

<Kung Fu Swish-Swish-Swish sound effect>

What to Do Next

Now that you've been strong-armed to comply, here is the best way to proceed. You'll need to make a list, so choose your favorite list-making material. Pen and paper. iThingamabob. Smoke signals. Whatever.

1. Make a list of all the vegetables and fruits you like.
2. Regardless of how long or short the list is, even if it's empty, add berries, broccoli, dark leafy greens, and at least one other cruciferous vegetables (see Food Lists Appendix for options). These foods are extremely nutrient-dense.
3. Place a #4, for mantra #4, next to all fruits (including the berries) and all starchy vegetables. If you don't know whether a vegetable is starchy or not, check out the Food Lists in the Appendix. Specific fruits that are neither sweet nor fruit-like, such as tomatoes and avocado, do not need the #4 next to them. They are vegetables as far as the plan is concerned.
4. Anything that doesn't have a #4 next to it is fair game to qualify for conforming to mantra #3.

For now, we are reserving fruits and starchy vegetables for the next mantra. These foods have relatively high carbohydrate content. Many people on *The Karma Sense Eating Plan* want to lose weight and need to watch carbs. That's why I've been saying "Vegetables and Fruits" and not "Fruits and Vegetables" like any rational human being. It's my way of asking you to put your emphasis on vegetables over fruits. When I discuss special considerations at the end of this chapter, I'll give you enough information so you know what to do. And, of course, you'll get more excruciating detail and other shenanigans in the next chapter as well. As a boss of mine once said, while channeling Yogi Berra, "patience comes to those who wait."

But What If I Don't Like What Remains?

Here are some thoughts on how to deal with this.

1. Don't try to reach seven to ten servings immediately. Build up to it. You may never get there. Yoda would say it's okay simply to try in this special case.
2. You've heard the expression "an acquired taste?" Perhaps you applied it to this book or you're hoping it may eventually be true about this book. It is a legitimate phenomenon recognized by flavor scientists. If you don't think flavor science exists, explain why anyone would ever eat anything that looks like a Hostess Sno-Ball.

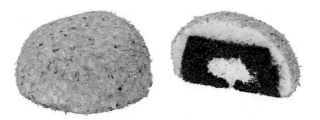

Figure 34 Hostess Sno-Ball. Now in Purple Flavor![105]

The theory of acquired taste is that you deem some aspect of the food unusual, and the only way to get over that is through more exposure. So don't dip your toe in the pool. Jump in all at once. You'll get used to it more quickly.
3. You've heard the expression "an unacquired taste?" Me neither. But we've both heard it now. It's possible to learn to dislike something that you really should because you had a bad

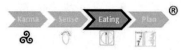

experience when you consumed it ("chicken roll cold cuts" did it for me although, to this day, I wonder why anyone would ever like them) or, more specifically, due to consistently bad preparation. For example, our parents had a lot on their plates. The last thing they needed to do was to clean, chop, season, and prepare your vegetables. Especially when there were such convenient versions available frozen or canned. Convenient? Yes. Tasty? Usually not. And so we unacquired any chance of liking vegetables. These days there are more convenient versions of fresh vegetables. They're already washed and chopped. And there are a million ways to sneak them into your diet, such as —

4. If you've never tried them raw, try them raw.

5. If you've never tried them cooked, try them cooked.

6. Chop them up fine and put them in your pasta sauce. Summer squash can even be used in place of pasta for a low-carb treat. There are recipes available for doing this that include some high-fallutin' sauces. But there's no reason you can't use a hearty spaghetti sauce. A powerfully flavored sauce works wonders for hiding flavors you think are yucky. Be careful though. Sauces can be tricky little calorie bombs with lots of hidden sugar or undesirable fat.

7. Cook them in an omelet.

8. Salad.

9. You can make mashed "potatoes," rice, and even pizza crust out of cauliflower. Google any of these or check out the Karma Sense Cooking section in the appendix for ideas.

10. My personal favorite. Roast them (suggestions in Karma Sense Cooking section of Appendix.) Roasting removes much of the bitterness people don't like and adds a crunchy, salty, fatty mouth feel that is akin to eating chips. Don't give up on this one. If you don't like the way it turns out with one vegetable, try another. Cauliflower and broccoli look a little alike, but their flavor, when roasted, is completely different. Cauliflower gets kind of sweet. Broccoli becomes more crispy/mild. Brussels

sprouts? I am the first to admit, there are few foods as heinous as an improperly prepared Brussels sprout. Roasted Brussels sprouts? Wow!

11. Turn it into a puzzle and figure out whatever the heck this is:

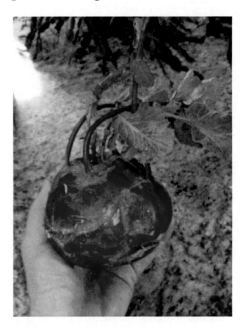

Figure 35 Kohlrabi - The Vegetable from Another Planet[106]

12. Eat asparagus. If you're childish as I am, trust me on this one. And if this appeals to you, you should read _Put It In Your Act_ by my pal Larry Osman.[107] You're in for a good time (heh heh).

13. Google for more ideas or just click here if you want to be lazy about it.[*]

14. ~~Spread them on your plate and hope no one notices them or feed them to the dog.~~

14. If all else fails, consider taking a greens supplement. The benefits are just too great to abandon.

---

[*] If reading the print version of the _Karma Sense Eating Plan_, do not bother clicking. Instead enter "what to do if people don't like vegetables" in your favorite internet search tool (which is what people in denial call "Google").

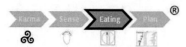

Special Considerations

This section explores how people with different goals should adjust the mantra of Eat More Vegetables and Fruits.

Lose Weight

Implement this mantra as is. Avoid starchy vegetables and fruits. Don't worry. You can be Karma Sensible, lose weight, and eat these, ahem, forbidden fruits. But do so according to mantra #4 to maximize weight loss.

Maintain Weight but Eat Healthier

Implement this mantra as is. Feel free to add the items on your list marked with the #4 next to them. Aim for a ratio of five servings of mantra #3 veggies to two servings from mantra #4.

Gain Weight in the Form of Muscle

Implement this mantra as is. This assumes you also have a significant exercise routine. If so, feel free to add #4s to your repertoire (which I believe is French for "stuff") but aim for less #4s than non-#4s, just because you like a challenge (no pain, no gain, Bro!).

Key Points

1. Eat seven to ten servings of vegetables and fruits per day.
2. A serving consists of:
   - One (1) cup green leafy vegetables
   - One (1) medium-sized piece of fruit
   - Half (½) cup chopped raw fruit, whole berries, or vegetables
3. Eating more plants is good Karma. It helps to save the world.
4. Aim to consume mostly cruciferous vegetables and dark leafy greens.

5. Eat starchy vegetables and fruits sparingly, although this may vary depending on your goals.

6. If you are one of the people who don't like vegetables, follow one of the many strategies for building a tolerance and even learning to love them.

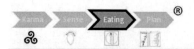

Karma Sense in the Wild

Some neighbors of mine used to enjoy giving me a hard time about my attempts to inflict my healthy lifestyle on my children. We'd be hanging around outside in the pre-dinner hour and inevitably the conversation would wander to what we're having for dinner. Ever since the time we answered "tofu" we became the culinary laughingstocks of our neighborhood. The joke was on them. At the time, our kids enjoyed tofu.

This was around the time that my sons and I underwent our transformation from "dad bods" to Greek Gods (your author is the exception from that latter category). Eventually the teasing stopped. Or at least it was reserved for when we weren't around. But one of our neighbors never let up. They had good health and maintained their health despite a dearth of vegetables in their diet. They just didn't like them.

Several years ago we moved to a new city in the same metropolitan area. We stayed in touch with some of our closest friends from the old hood and that included the veggie-haters. We recently went out to dinner and I ordered my current obsession, roasted Brussels sprouts (Ben & Jerry's Chubby Hubby wasn't on the menu). It turned out that the chief instigator of my ridicule recently became fond of this crack-like vegetable preparation herself. I asked them whether broccoli was also on their menu and they said it was something they could now tolerate. I suggested they try roasting them just like they do with Brussels sprouts? They said they'd give it a try.

I checked in with these folks a few months later to ask them if they tried it. It turns out the broccoli recommendation was pretty clutch. While mom remains a fan of Brussels sprouts, the rest of the family doesn't like the way the house smells. Broccoli is a different story. They add a little lemon to the oil and it's now one of their sons' favorite foods. Two adolescent boys are requesting broccoli!

If you don't Eat Vegetables in Every Meal because you don't like them, don't give up. Your health, happiness, and world-saving skills depend upon it. Your taste buds deserve it.

Mantra #4: Eat Whole Food Carbohydrates After Vigorous Exercise

Executive Summary

We're on the home stretch of the Eating component. This chapter covers mantra #4, Eat Whole Food Carbohydrates After Vigorous Exercise. The usual stuff is covered here. What? How Much? When? And everyone's favorite, why?

We have a lot of learning to do, so please report to...

Home Room

We need to begin with a few announcements.

While the subject of carbohydrates should be simple, it's quite complex (LOL! Nutritionist humor!). Several cliques would love to control your relationship with carbohydrates. Many of our decisions on how to deal with carbohydrates are based on peer pressure (both overt and subtle). And the biggest drivers of how we should eat and process carbs are hormones.

Hmmm, cliques? Peer pressure? Hormones? Sounds like high school. So in that spirit,

Ring, Ring. Time to go to first period.

English Class

Beowulf, The Scarlet Letter, The Canterbury Tales. You probably remember these like it was yesterday. Me? I remember the titles and only because they sound like things I'd read about in comic books. Although I do remember "The Miller's Tale" portion of *The Canterbury Tales* very well. Wonder why that one lingers?

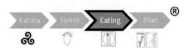

Anyway, dig a little deeper into that memory. Do you recall there were five major conflict-oriented themes to look for when reading great literature? If not, here's a reminder:

1. Man vs. Man
2. Man vs. Himself
3. Man vs. Society
4. Man vs. Nature
5. Man vs. Giant Nuclear Monsters Whose Purpose in Life is to Trash Tokyo

Coincidentally, almost as if it was planned (but I assure you nothing around here is), these same conflicts can be found in the writings of *The Karma Sense Eating Plan*. For example, mantra #2, Eat Protein in Every Meal, is a sassy tale about the disagreement among nutrition experts who still debate the amount of protein we should eat at the expense of other macronutrients. Yet they totally ignore that the reputable experts agree more than they disagree and that their back-and-forth confuses the rest of us. It's your classic Man vs. Man.

Mantra #3, Eat More Vegetables and Fruits, discusses the conflict we have within ourselves. The angel on our right shoulder whispers in our ear that we should eat the succotash on our plate. That devil on the left says, "Gee, the dog looks kind of hungry. Hey Mom, look over there!" It's Man vs. Himself.

What about mantra #4, Eat Whole Food Carbohydrates After Vigorous Exercise? Much to our mutual chagrin, this mantra is not an example of Man vs. Giant Nuclear Monsters Whose Purpose in Life is to Trash Tokyo. That would be silly. Godzilla is pure protein. Our conflict is Man vs. Society. It's a society that sells and subsidizes highly refined carbohydrates in a manner not too different from the way the kid in the boys room peddles dope. It's a society where nuance and subtlety are not appreciated and drives everyone to extremes. And, it's a society that is split between those who view carbs as something that can never be enjoyed responsibly and those who can't imagine a meal without them.

So what is the lesson from today's class?

1. Because *The Karma Sense Eating Plan* evokes these classic themes, it's apparently a great piece of literature after all. Maybe even right up there with Faulkner's *Absalom, Absalom!* because it's another piece of writing most people can't figure out.
2. Outside interests drive our relationship with carbohydrates. It is an individual's job to "make peace" with the relationship that works best.

Ring, Ring. Time to go to second period.

History Class

Today's lesson covers the longest war ever fought. It's still underway to this day. It is a war among loosely knit tribes, and it has a lasting effect on our relationship with carbohydrates. The tribes are led by:

1. The Tasty-But-Empty-Calorie Cabal whose strength lies in a never-ending supply of money.
2. The Healthy Lifestyle Militia who, through their extreme and convincing positions, elevate their fame and fortune.
3. The (Karma) Sensible Revolutionaries, a loose-knit rag-tag bunch who look out for our best interests. Unfortunately, the Revolutionaries are the underdogs.
4. House Baratheon.

Here is the background that led to this war.

Ever since the first man and woman ignored a perfectly good portion of reptile protein and snake oil (mantras #2 and #5, respectively) for an apple, carbohydrates have been a source of temptation, shame, and guilt. (Wait. Are we sure it was an apple? A donut seems to make more sense to me. I can't imagine anyone ever feeling guilty about an apple.)

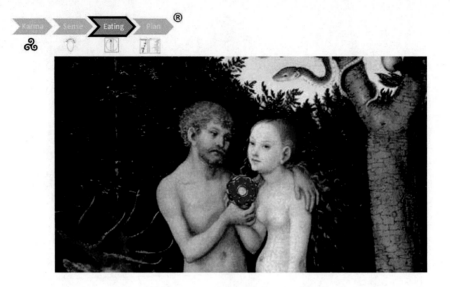

Figure 36 And on the Eighth Day, the Lord Kreated Krispy Kreme and Boy Was it Good.[108]

As the human race continued to grow, our ancestors ate whatever was available. What was available was a bunch of plants and the occasional tasty creature. Some of those creatures returned our hungry glances because they thought our predecessors looked delicious. This left little time or patience for preparing and digesting food. People ate grains sparingly since they required lots of prep work. Let me say that again with some specific emphasis for modern followers of the Paleo lifestyle. Ancient people *ate* grains sparingly.

On the other hand, foods like fruits were coveted (as long as they were not thy neighbor's), because the sweet taste told our brains, "You're about to get a quick hit of vital energy."

Eventually, we went from hunter-gatherer to farmer-consumer. The management and accessibility of our nutrition became easier. The wealthy ate what they wanted. The poor ate what was left. As cities started to emerge and the middle-class gained expendable income, the wealthy learned that, if they could make their leftovers more appealing to the masses, they could raise demand and create better profit margins. And so, through the wonders of chemistry and other sciences, they found cheap ways to make bad food taste better. And this is how the first tribe, a well-organized cabal of food processors, advertisers, media companies, and middle men, was formed. It was a Tasty-But-Empty-Calorie Cabal (these guys show up later in this story as they find more allies in their midst.)

As a society, we were unsophisticated, which allowed commercials like the one depicted in the scene below and at this link. The ad uses two characters from the popular live-action *"Superman"* show to push a highly refined grain and sugar concoction as "part of a healthy breakfast." The rest of the "healthy" breakfast included fruit juice (with the fiber removed and sometimes with added sugar) and jelly (fruit with added sugar) on white toast (with added sugar). Some people even added sugar to the bowl of cereal.

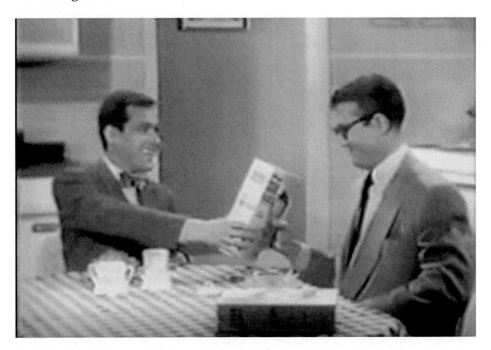

Figure 37 This is a manly breakfast we're sharing, Mr. Kent.[109,110]

The commercial's premise is that Jimmy Olsen and Clark Kent are about to sit down for breakfast when Jimmy notices they're out of cereal. In

---

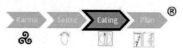

response, Clark ducks away and changes into Superman so he can quickly fly to get more. Once more, Superman saves the day.

Golly, if Superman eats corn flakes, they must be good for you, right? And while most people pondered that question, I was thinking:

1. Does Clark Kent keep a phone booth in his house so he can change into his Superman costume?
2. When he gets to the supermarket, does he have to change back into his Clark Kent outfit?
3. If so, where does he keep it?
4. If not, where does he keep his wallet?
5. Or does SuperMAN shop at a special SuperMARKET?

In the end, that specific commercial isn't so misleading since all it really says is, "Be like Superman and eat cornflakes." But by choosing this ad as an example, I get to include a superhero reference and that makes me happy. It also allows me to go on a tangent that I'll somehow tie back to the subject at hand.

Kellogg's sponsored the *Superman* show and had many commercials that included the show's stars. Sometimes Jimmy Olsen was replaced by Perry White. But Lois Lane never got a piece of the sweet endorsement cash. This wasn't due to the glass ceiling at work, at least not directly. It was because Kellogg's sold breakfast food and thought it would be too racy for Lois and Clark to be sharing breakfast.[111]

These days, advertisers have no problem referencing sexy-time. They get more scrutiny for pushing junk food as healthful. This change only came about because of the subtle yet hamstrung influence of the (Karma) Sensible Revolutionaries in an attempt to keep the Tasty-But-Empty-Calorie Cabal accountable. Now instead of making specious health claims, the Cabal resorts to peer pressure, telling us that TGI Frapplebees is a fun place to watch the game, has the tastiest candy-apple-chicken-wings at the strip mall and you'll definitely get laid if you go.

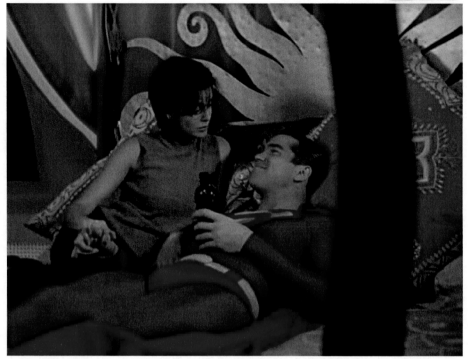

Figure 38 Welcome to My Fortress of Product Placement and Solitude.[112,113]

Meanwhile, a contingency of people began to cherry-pick the results of well-meaning research and turn them into easily consumable attacks on the Tasty-But-Empty-Calorie Cabal. Some did this with the best intentions. Many did it purely to chip away at the big pile of dough made by the Cabal. For example, the mostly discredited low-fat movement began with an ignorant yet noble purpose. It also happened to make wads of cash for vendors of low-fat products, including the only thing more unnatural, horrible, and destructive than Giant Nuclear Monsters Whose Purpose in Life is to Trash Tokyo. Yes, I'm talking about fat-free salad dressing. Thus, the genesis of The Healthy Lifestyle Militia.

The Militia's leaders include Paleo-Zealots, Anti-Gluteneers, and Bulletproof Extremists. I'd be the first to say, much of what The Militia preaches would be Karma Sensible if they didn't deal in absolutes

---

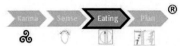

("Never eat grains. They're poison for all!"). When it comes to a nutrition plan that is healthful and sustainable, there is no one-size-fits-all solution. And the beat goes on.

Throughout all this, the (Karma) Sensible Revolutionaries persevere and evangelize moderation in all things. Much like the soldiers in the American Revolution, these warriors are underdogs. They lack funding. They lack data (given that the Cabal sponsors more and more health research and expects a predetermined outcome). They lack the ability to get attention (moderation is dull). What they have is the truth. That's a powerful weapon.

Every day this war is fought right in front of our eyes. We watch a (Karma) Sensible Revolutionary featured in a segment on the news followed by a Cabal sponsored commercial break for flavored sugar water, medications to help control Type 2 Diabetes, and previews for the next episode of *The Biggest Loser* starring members of The Militia.

And that's the story of the longest war ever fought. So what is the lesson from today's class?

1. The author of *The Karma Sense Eating Plan* is intent on weaving superhero references into everything he does.
2. A huge fight for your attention and money exists where food is concerned. Don't fall victim to the loudest or most persistent voice.

Ring, Ring. Time to go to third period.

Latin Class
Ood-gay orning-may, ass-clay. Epeat-ray After-yay E-may
[*Good morning class. Repeat after me.*]

E-thay Arma-Kay Ense-Say Eating-yay An-Play is-yay inclusive-yay.
[*The Karma Sense Eating Plan is inclusive.*]

It-yay is-yay esigned-day o-tay ake-may you-yay ealthier-hay, appier-hay, and-yay, oh-yay yeah-yay, ave-say e-thay orld-way.
[It is designed to make you healthier, happier, and, oh yeah, save the world.]

Very good. Now for the rest of class, proceed to what you usually do despite the assignment — research how to curse in a foreign language.

Ring, Ring. Before progressing to fourth period, a brief announcement.

1. Will the owner of the red Oldsmobile Alero please remove your car from the parking lot? It has not moved in months and is a neighborhood eyesore.
2. Will the writer of this chapter please get to the point for people who just want to know what to do to honor mantra #4?

Yes, but he'll do so during fourth period,

Linguistics Class - Elective

Today class we're going to parse a very dense and succinct statement, *Eat Whole Food Carbohydrates After Vigorous Exercise.*

Eat

Something to do slowly and stop doing before you're full.

Whole Food

Whole food in this sense means minimally (or better yet, not) processed. So you can put away your wallets. I'm not talking about the upscale supermarket (a perfectly fine institution). Do you remember how "processed" was so scientifically defined in mantra #2, Eat Protein in Every Meal? Our definition for this mantra is a little tighter. Pay close attention to the number and types of ingredients. The fewer the better. All of these ingredients should be real food. For example, ingredients for a box of pasta should consist of no more than whole grain flour, water, salt, and egg. But be wary. Many of these "healthy" options contain

---

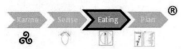

maltodextrin or corn syrup (which are Tasty-But-Empty-Calorie Cabal terms for "sugar"). Your best bet is to buy foods that aren't required to label ingredient (i.e., fresh and raw).

Carbohydrates

We defer the propeller head discussion of *Carbohydrates* for science class (Oh yes, there will be a science class). For the purposes of linguistics, we mean:

- Beans, lentils, and other legumes
- The starchy vegetables that you labeled with #4's on the list you created for mantra #3. Didn't make a list? Refer to the list of starchy vegetables in the Appendix, Food Lists.
- Fruit
- Grains in their whole, unprocessed form

A few things to note about this list. The higher up the list, the more I encourage you to select that choice. Yes, legumes are on the protein list, too. But they're starchy-carby protein (a.k.a., carb-olicious). They're essential for vegetarians, soul food for many cultures, and a great side dish for meat eaters. That's also why they are the most preferred whole food carbohydrate.

Starchy vegetables are only slightly ahead of fruit. The reason involves a whole 'nother (what the heck is a 'nother, anyway?) tangent about how the predominant sugar in fruit, fructose, is processed in the liver. But this is *The Karma Sense Eating Plan* after all, so do what you want. Who am I to judge?

Grains such as rice, barley, and wheat are perfectly Karma Sensible. I am not a Militia extremist who believes grains are the root of all evil including our obesity epidemic, Type 2 Diabetes, and the cancellation of the TV program *Firefly* (hey, it was a good show).

The Karma Sense Eating Plan does have a place for refined carbohydrates. It's just not part of mantra #4. Believe me, any plan that won't support my habit of honoring the original sin of eating a donut or participating in the Ben & Jerry Chubby Hubby Desert Island Experiment (see mantra #3, Eat More Vegetables and Fruits) is not a plan I can endorse. By the way, many people don't know this, but refined carbohydrates are called refined because they're made in a refinery (a.k.a., factory). They're not called refined because they have sophisticated behaviors such as avoiding vomiting all over their prom dates. True story.

Alcohol is a whole 'nother kettle of fish (not literally a kettle of fish) that I discuss in the Appendix, Alcohol and Its Role in Karma Sense Eating.

After

By after we mean within two hours after finishing exercise. Not before. During would be messy. More than a couple of hours is right out. (It's like counting to five with the Holy Hand Grenade from *Monty Python and the Holy Grail*.)

This time limit may seem a little too specific for *The Karma Sense Eating Plan* and indeed it is. We'll discuss this further during Science class (oh yes, there will be a science class). It's much less strict yet more nuanced than it currently appears.

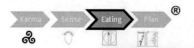

> And the LORD spake, saying,
> "First shalt thou take out the Holy Pin,
> then shalt thou count to three,
> no more, no less.
> Three shall be the number thou shalt count,
> and the number of the counting shall be three.
> Four shalt thou not count,
> neither count thou two,
> excepting that thou then proceed to three.
> Five is right out.
> Once the number three, being the third number,
> be reached, then lobbest thou
> thy Holy Hand Grenade of Antioch
> towards thy foe, who being naughty in My sight,
> shall snuff it. - Book of Armaments

Figure 39 Instructions for the Holy Hand Grenade.[114,115]

Vigorous Exercise

We'll parse this part of the mantra during what else?

Ring, Ring. Time to go to fifth period.

Physical Education (PE) Class

Let's go over the specifics of "vigorous exercise." But first let's note that these exercises are for moderately healthy and active people. If you're not quite in this category, you need to work up to it first. If you're beyond that category, you probably don't need to reserve your carbohydrates until after exercise. Regardless, check with your health support team before engaging in any significantly new activity (e.g., check with your doctor if you haven't been exercising at all and want to run an Ironman. Not to be confused with the superhero.).

The term *vigorous exercise* is nebulous and subject to much interpretation. For the sake of hanging our hat somewhere, we'll go with the US Centers for Disease Control <u>definition</u>.[116] Based on this, intensity can be measured using one of the following:

- The *talk test* is a simple way to measure relative intensity. In general, if you're doing moderate-intensity activity, you can talk but not sing. If you're doing vigorous activity, you will not be able to say more than a few words without pausing for a breath. If you can sing while doing physical activity, your intensity is light. Even though light activity isn't vigorous, don't let that stop you from singing. *The Karma Sense Eating Plan* is all about making you healthy, saving the world, and oh yeah, making you happy. <u>Studies</u> show that singing leads to happiness.[117,118,119] So go ahead and sing. Sing the theme from Spiderman or from Batman. Heck, you don't even have to sing TV superhero themes. I've never tried, but I bet other songs would make you happy too.
- For a relative scale, assign a number based on your relative fitness on a scale of zero to ten where zero is no effort and ten is 100% all out sprint. Vigorous physical activity is usually a seven or eight.

Vigorous activities tend to include:

- Race walking, jogging, and running
- Swimming laps
- Tennis (singles)
- Aerobic dancing
- Bicycling ten miles per hour or faster
- Jumping rope
- Dodge Ball vs. the 1985 Chicago Bears (as long as it's 1985)
- Heavy gardening (continuous digging or hoeing. No comments from you jokers in the back.)
- Hiking uphill or with a heavy backpack
- Escaping from Tokyo as it is being trashed by Giant Nuclear Monsters.

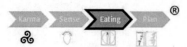

Because *The Karma Sense Eating Plan* is all about giving and not taking away, it includes moderately intense resistance exercise such as weight training and body weight exercises.

Finally, there's the question of duration. Ideal is fifteen to thirty minutes of the vigorous exercises listed above before indulging in carbohydrates. Are you moderately healthy and don't have thirty minutes? Try following the routine discussed in the Appendix, Don't Waste Your Time Exercising.

And that is it for today.

Civil, instructive, well-organized, and no bruises—that's how you remember your PE class, right?

Ring, Ring. Time for...

Lunch

Today's special is one to two servings of protein with two to three servings of vegetables over whole-grain pasta (It's OK, you just had a vigorous game of Dodge Ball in PE) in a sauce of healthy fat. Mmmm. Don't forget to honor your good deed, the good deeds of others, and the efforts of those fine cafeteria workers behind the counter. Enjoy your lunch slowly, and stop before you're full.

Ring, Ring. Was that twenty minutes already? Time flies when you're eating slowly. Time to go to sixth period.

Biology Class

(I bet you weren't expecting a science class.)

Your body's metabolism of carbohydrates is unique compared to protein and fats. Carbs follow different pathways depending on what you ate, when you ate it, and your own individual physiology. These different pathways have a direct effect on your health. To appreciate this fully requires a level of geekiness that even I'm uncomfortable inflicting upon you. But, if you want to manage your Karma Sense Eating without support from a coach, I need to go into some detail. I promise, I'll only tell you what you need to know, but I may go astray to make a wiseacre remark. This explanation may err on the side of oversimplification. Nutrition pedants, I'm ready to suffer the consequences but please be civil.

The Science of "Eat Whole Food Carbohydrates"

As soon as your food enters your mouth, saliva begins to break carbs into their simplest form, sugar. As the food continues through your digestive tract, more of the carbs are converted into simple sugar. Once the food reaches the small intestines, some, but not all carbs, transfer to your blood stream. The portion that *is not* transferred continues through your digestive tract and is removed from the body (use your imagination). The undigested portion was just checking out the sights; passing through.

The carbs that *are* absorbed continue to the liver which acts as a factory and distribution warehouse. The liver keeps some of the sugar and circulates the rest onto the nutrition superhighway, your bloodstream. The circulating sugar is stored in a variety of places:

1. A couple teaspoons circulate in the blood and are used for quick energy and to feed the brain because unlike other cells in the body, brain cells can't store their own energy. But the blood can only hold so much sugar in it before turning into syrup. Your body likes to keep your blood at a pre-syrup level. So, it stashes the sugar in other places such as…
2. Your liver and muscle tissue where the sugar is used for energy. But the liver and muscles can only store so much. If the liver and muscles are full, and there's no more room at the inn, the sugar converts to
3. Fat.

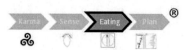

One strategy to minimize the amount of sugar stored as fat is to maximize your intake of whole food carbohydrates instead of simpler, refined carbs. Simple carbohydrates, like refined sugars and flours, are absorbed very efficiently. Complex carbohydrates which have lots of fiber, are more of a challenge to the digestive system. The digestive system truly loves a challenge, but it doesn't do as well processing the foods that present the challenge. That's good news because you experience all the enjoyment of eating an entire sweet potato without it having the same metabolic effect as eating the equivalent amount of SweetTARTS. This is why mantra #4 emphasizes Whole Food Carbohydrates instead of their refined cousins. Note that the Tasty-But-Empty-Calorie Cabal is always interested in finding new names and cheaper techniques to provide sugar. Here are some examples to look for on an ingredient label:

A Small Sample of the Many Names for "Sugar"		
Agave Nectar	Glucose	Maltose
Sugar	High Fructose Corn Syrup	Maltodextrin
Corn Syrup	Hydrolyzed Starch	Maple Syrup
Dextrose	Honey	Molasses
Fruit Juice	Hubby, Chubby	Sucrose
Fructose	Inverted Sugar Syrup	Sugar Beets

Table 6 Sugar by Any Other Name Will Taste as Sweet

These ingredients are not carbohydrates in the spirit of mantra #4. Fear not, if you have a jones for hydrolyzed starch (and who doesn't?), it's time will come when we describe the Plan component .

The Science of "After Vigorous Exercise"

If we consider the three ways the body stores carbohydrates and assume you want to minimize the third (i.e., fat), we have two main strategies. The first is to manage the type of carbs you eat (complex, whole foods; not simple nor refined). The second is to manage the timing of when you eat them. Here is the theory of operations for the timing.

Fat and muscle cells absorb much of the sugar sent to the blood by the liver. The exceptions are sugar that's immediately used for fuel and to maintain blood sugar levels. Sugar enters fat and muscle cells through a series of pumps called Glucose Transporters that pull the sugar from the blood, enabling it to enter the cells. One specific Glucose Transporter, called GLUT4, pumps sugar into muscle and fat cells. Our goal is to pack as much sugar as possible into the muscle cells and not the fat cells. However, GLUT4s are shy. They don't welcome sugar at all hours of the day and night. If they did, they would be GLUT-10s (which, I admit, is a very bad joke). Instead, they depend on either (or both) of two events:

1. Insulin Release - Insulin is a hormone (at last, those promised hormones) secreted by the pancreas when the liver has no choice but to push all the extra sugar it's received into the bloodstream. In the presence of insulin, your muscles and fat cells activate your GLUT4s to pull sugar from the blood and store it in their cells. The amount of sugar that can be stored relates directly to how much muscle and fat tissue you have. Once we're adults, we only gain new muscle when we use our muscles in new and challenging ways. Unfortunately, we gain fat simply by taking in more calories than we burn. This means muscle has an upper limit on how much sugar it can store. Fat does not. And the more sugar stored in your fat, the more fat you carry around. If you consume too much sugar over your lifetime, you may become insulin resistant. This is like the ding-dong-ditch of bodily

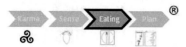

functions. Your cells get so tired of insulin knocking on the door that they stop sending GLUT4s to answer. The sugar circulates in the blood and lines your cell walls with candy coating like an M&M. This is a condition known as Type 2 Diabetes.

2. Vigorous Exercise - When you exercise, your muscle cells use stored sugar for energy. They do this through a complicated system called the Krebs Cycle which, contrary to popular belief, is not named after Maynard G. Krebs of the once popular television program, *The Many Loves of Dobie Gillis.*

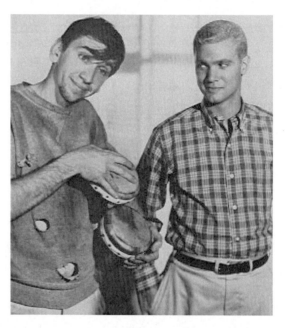

Figure 40 Maynard G. Krebs (on left) and Dobie Gillis[120,121]

In fact, the Krebs Cycle isn't critical to this discussion at all. But, Maynard G. Krebs? He's just a hip cat. But back to vigorous exercise. As the stored sugar is consumed, muscle cells engage the GLUT4s to pull in more sugar. This optimizes the amount of sugar targeted for muscles. Fat cells do not need to engage their GLUT4s during exercise because fat isn't doing any work. Also, if you work hard enough and follow mantra #2, Eat Protein in

Every Meal, your muscles will grow, and that means they can take on more sugar next time.

And this is why, for mantra #4, you Eat Whole Food Carbohydrates After Vigorous Exercise. Whole Food Carbs because they don't get absorbed as sugar as easily. After Vigorous Exercise because this maximizes uptake in the muscle and minimizes the addition of fat.

So what is the lesson from today's class?

1. Admit it, science really was the best class you ever had, and you actually do use it in real life.
2. If your goal is optimal health, the type of carbs and the timing of when you eat them matters.

Ring, Ring. Time to go to seventh (and final) period.

Math Class

Today's class will cover everyone's favorite activity—word problems. The problems focus on adding enough carbs in the diet. It is important to note that active people need more carbs than people who are sedentary. The topics below apply mostly to active folk.

- Maynard is fit, active, and does not really crave carbohydrates. He learned in school that carbs can make him fat. He figures he'll just stop eating them. How many words are required to explain to Maynard why long-term avoidance of carbs is a bad idea? *Solution:* One. And that word is "hormones" (there they are again).
- Davey H is pushing his luck with this chapter if he expects us to read something this long. For planning purposes, how many hormonal problems will he tell us about? **Extra credit for listing the affected hormones and the associated issue.** *Solution:* Seven.

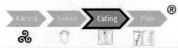

#	Hormone	Purpose	Issue
1	T3	Thyroid hormone increases metabolism, regulates bone growth, ensures proper neural development and drives your body's ability to process protein.	Insufficient carbohydrate intake lowers availability of T3 to the body. (study[122])
2	Testosterone	Secreted by the sex glands of both men and women, its effects are not restricted solely to "mojo." Besides being a key component of sexy-time, it's a critical hormone for muscle development, fat loss, bone health and overall performance for both sexes.	Prolonged low carb diets are linked to drops in testosterone levels. (study[123])
3	Estrogen	These are (primarily) female sex hormones critical to an exhaustive list of women's health functions that I won't get into because your parents haven't signed the waiver.	Women seem especially vulnerable to sustained low-carbohydrate intake which causes a reduction in these critical hormones. The disruption actually happens earlier in the sequence of events that drive hormone production, but I'll spare you the details. (study[124])
4	Progesterone		
5	Follicle Stimulating Hormone		
6	Luteinizing Hormone		
7	Cortisol	A multifunction adrenal hormone. Cortisol is a hormone that allows your body to respond to stress.	Prolonged low-carb diets cause chronic elevation in cortisol which leads to increased inflammation (bad), decreased muscle tone, and increased fat storage, especially in the belly. (study[125])

Table 7 Hormone Issues Related to Insufficient Carbohydrate Intake.

- Batman, Wonder Woman, Spiderman, and Jean Gray are having a dinner party ninety minutes after working out in the X-Men's Danger Room. They will have a whole grain pasta side dish. How many servings should they prepare? What size are the portions? *Solution:* Trick Question. These four are from different comic universes. It would be impossible for them to meet. Furthermore, of all the macronutrients, carbs may be the hardest to fit into a one size fits all response for daily consumption. As a rule of thumb, start with half a cup of cooked whole food carbohydrates for women and one cup for men. The actual answer depends on many variables including:
  - Physiology - some people are more carb tolerant or process carbs more efficiently than others.
  - Activity level - active people need more carbohydrates than sedentary people.
  - Goals - people looking to lose weight can opt for a lower-carbohydrate diet than people looking to maintain or gain weight.
- Some readers are interested in figuring out the right serving size for them. How do they proceed?
  Solution: Trial and error mostly. Start with the above guidelines and adjust accordingly. There are other ways to pinpoint right amounts, but they are beyond the scope of this course. I am happy to stay after class and discuss this. Please <u>contact me</u>* if interested. At the end of the day, which thankfully we have now reached, don't over-think it. Relax. Use the Force.

Ring, Ring. The school day is done. Here are some things to consider.

---

* Email: <u>daveyh@livelongleadlong.com</u>; Twitter: @LiveAndLeadLong;
Facebook: <u>http://www.facebook.com/livelongleadlong</u>

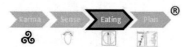

Special Considerations

Time to explore how people with different goals should adjust the mantra of Eat Whole Food Carbohydrates After Vigorous Exercise.

Lose Weight

Implement this mantra as is. If you're deferring or declining the adoption of Mantra #2, Eat Protein in Every Meal, be sure to at least eat protein after vigorous exercise. Your body needs it in order to recover and prevent muscle breakdown. If you find you're not losing weight, you might consider deferring all carbohydrates for a little while.

Maintain Weight but Eat Healthier

Implement this mantra as is. If you're inclined to explore the limits, go ahead and let us know how it works out for you. Breakfast is a good meal to test first. When you first wake up, you're in a fasted state. The needle on your stored and circulating sugar gauge is pushing towards empty. Breaking your fast with whole food carbs (e.g., oatmeal; not Chocolate Crunchy Sugar Bombs) is a good way to refill your tank. Your body depends on the insulin mechanism for engaging your GLUT4s (described in Biology class) which means muscle and fat cells will take up the available sugar. But if the rest of your diet makes Karma sense, don't expect it to affect your weight.

If you're deferring or declining adoption of Mantra #2, Eat Protein in Every Meal, be sure to at least eat protein after vigorous exercise. Your body needs it in order to recover and prevent muscle breakdown.

Gain Weight in the Form of Muscle

You have more leeway to implement this. For example, feel free to add some fruit to your regular meals. Be sure to eat some protein after vigorous exercise too. You probably will not gain muscle if you don't recover with protein.

Key Points

1. The subject of carbohydrates and your consumption of them is complicated, highly individualized, and made more confusing by outside sources and forces. Don't let these get to you. Common sense will serve you well. Karma Sense will serve you better.

2. Aim for minimally processed sources of carbohydrates in the following order of preference (highest to lowest):
   - Beans, lentils, and other legumes
   - The starchy vegetables that you labeled with #4's on the list you created for mantra #3.
   - Fruit
   - Whole Grains

3. Other carbohydrates, including those that are highly refined (flour based or added sugar) and alcohol (not really a carb), are not included in mantra #4. They are discussed later in the book.

4. Eat whole food carbohydrates within two hours after vigorous exercise. Vigorous means:
   - You can't speak more than a few words without taking a breath. Vigorous also means about a seven or eight on a relative difficulty scale where ten means all-out effort.
   - Instead of the above, you can participate in moderate resistance exercise such as weight training.

5. Aim for at least fifteen to thirty minutes of physical activity.

6. Portion sizes can vary and require monitoring based on your goals. For starters, a woman should go for half a cup cooked whole food carb. A man should go for one cup whole food carb. Both can be replaced by one medium piece of fruit or half a cup of whole berries/chopped fruit.

7. Eat Whole Food Carbs because they don't absorb quickly. Do so After Vigorous Exercise because it maximizes sugar uptake in the muscle and minimizes the addition of fat.

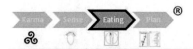

Karma Sense in the Wild

Doug is my age and he's totally ripped. Not steroid-infused professional wrestler ripped, more like triathlete ripped. Doug's a really easy guy to get to know. He's friendly and upbeat. If you ask him "How're you doing?" he never gives the same answer twice but it's always buoyant and personal. Optimistic declarations like his make sense as research consistently demonstrates their positive effect on the mood and outlook of certain people.[126]

Doug attributes some of his positive attitude to a decision he made many years ago. He's a vegetarian. He decided to give up meat after working on a cattle farm one summer. As he got to know the cows and their mates, it really put a damper on his enthusiasm for the drive thru window. His ability to succeed at vegetarianism was a boost to his self-esteem and, as the aforementioned study shows, positive self statements work better for people with high self-esteem.

To me the amazing thing is that a guy who avoids protein in its most efficient form could have such enviable muscle tone. Doug became a vegetarian in his late teens when it's much easier for a man to build muscle. It's hard work to build muscle when you're middle aged but it's not as hard to maintain it if it's already there (said your author, regretting his years as a desk-bound couch potato).

Lately though, Doug is starting to feel his body change. This no doubt is related to getting a little older. However, he's also noticing it as he regains interest in competing in the triatholons he used to love. He's sluggish and he believes he's a little more jiggly than he used to be. Most of us would be happy being twice as jiggly.

Doug's perception, however, is believable. Studies show that as we age, our bodies change in ways that affect digestion and absorption of all nutrients, including carbohydrates.[127] It's possible that these changes are leading to the sluggish feeling and the perceived bloat. We talked about his diet and I learned that it's been stable for years. He gets most of his protein from soy, a little dairy, and other plant-based sources, many of which are high in carbohydrates. He fills out his meals with vegetables, fruits, and whole grains.

I sought permission to give Doug some advice and he agreed. That advice was that he should Eat Whole Food Carbohydrates After Vigorous Exercise. This is more challenging for vegetarian athletes since so many of their options are carb-olicious. Some of his choices though were mostly carbs (e.g. pasta, quinoa, bread). He agreed to try limiting these foods to periods shortly after he exercised.

I caught up with Doug a few weeks later. He said he definitely felt more energetic. This could be the placebo effect but there's nothing wrong with that. The placebo effect is not a bad thing (if it works, it's almost always a better solution than drugs or other medical procedures). Doug also said that he lost a few pounds and it felt to him that it was where he felt most jiggly. There are a number of reasons why this may be so. It could be the GLUT-4 mechanism doing its job. I suspect it's also that he is eating fewer carbs in general. By timing his carb intake as he has, he's probably lost some water weight in the process and reduced his overall carbohydrate consumption. He's getting the results he wants even if it isn't through the process we expect.

That's the cool thing about *The Karma Sense Eating Plan.* It asks you to do certain things based on well-known scientific facts on how the human body works. But things don't always work the way they do in the lab. It doesn't matter. Sometimes the end justifies the means. Sometimes the means justifies the end. Even if it gets you there in a way you didn't expect.

Mantra #5: Eat Good Fats Daily and Balance a Variety of Good Fats

Executive Summary

This chapter focuses on the fifth and final mantra of the Eating component, Eat Good Fats Daily and Balance a Variety of Good Fats. This mantra should be a breath of fresh air after the complexity of mantra #4, Eat Whole Food Carbohydrates After Vigorous Exercise. It's quite simple to manage. Timing isn't a consideration. And everyone loves fat. It is a superior vehicle for delivering flavor and texture to food. Yet somehow we so-called nutrition experts managed to muck it up. And we had help. This chapter will right these wrongs.

For now, let's tell a little story. It's sort of embarrassing so let's just say it's a story about a "friend."

A "Friend"

This "friend" was a shy, awkward, funny looking kid, but he seemed to get along OK. When he got a little older, somehow, a nasty rumor about him circulated in school. It doesn't matter what the rumor was because it was just baseless gossip and repeating it only perpetuates the lie. But it was clever gossip because it weaved in aspects of my friend that were totally true and believable. He was shunned. Outcast. Banished. No reindeer games for him. Persona non grata (which I believe is Pig Latin for Nperso non tgra). You get the idea.

It was a pity. He was a nice kid. He was helpful and considerate. He had his friends' backs. He had a lot going for him.

So my friend ended up spending a lot of time alone. He didn't go out much. He developed some very unhealthy habits. Eventually, because he was a good guy, he began to hang out with a different crowd, certainly not the cool kids. But around his new crew, he was popular. And he thrived. Thrived to the point where the in-crowd started to notice. Little

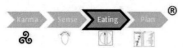

by little, they began inviting him into their circle. New rumors started to circulate, but they were about how awesome he was. He got swept up in his new popularity and ignored his old crew. It wasn't that he didn't like them. He just didn't have time for them anymore.

Eventually, the guy who had been so devastated by the negative rumors started to bask in the new positive ones. He was becoming a hero (but fear not, dear reader, no superheroes in this story). Then, one day, an emergency happened amongst the popular kids. It was one that only my friend with his rumored and fully imagined awesomeness could fix. But that awesomeness was fake. There was no way he or anyone else could help.

Through dumb luck that had nothing to do with my friend, disaster was averted. But now everyone knew he was a fraud. He was sent to the penalty box. Meanwhile, his old crew had moved on. Once again my friend became a loner.

Fortunately, he had college to look forward to; a chance to begin anew with all those lessons learned and the added benefit of still being a nice kid who was helpful and considerate and really had his friends' back.

And do you know what happened to my friend? Do you?

He was swept up and eaten by a Giant Nuclear Monster while visiting Tokyo. That's because my friend is totally made-up (it should come as no surprise that most of my friends are imaginary).

This story is 5% me, 20% *Mean Girls*, 10% *Rudolph the Red Nose Reindeer*, 20% *Peggy Sue Got Married*, 10% from the *Seinfeld* episode when George pretends to be a marine biologist, and the rest from just about every other teen angst movie ever written.

While the story is fiction, it pretty much mirrors the real-life story of fat as a part of a healthful diet. The rest of this chapter discusses the role of fat in the diet, the kind of fat we should seek out, how much we should eat, and some of the things we should look for as we honor mantra #5. However, to be fair to those who just want to know what to do and then be left alone, here are the particulars about mantra #5.

Eat Good Fats Daily and Balance a Variety of Good Fats

To understand the essence of this mantra, we need to establish the different fat categories. We also need to distinguish between good fats and bad fats. The easiest way to do this is with a table:

| Type | Saturated | Polyunsaturated | | Monounsa-turated | Trans fat |
		Omega-3	Omega-6		
Source	Animal fats, tropical oils such as coconut	Fish, algae, some nuts and seeds	Vege-table oils, many nuts and seeds	Olive oil, avocado, many nuts and seeds	Innocent scientists who were kidnapped by shell corpora-tions created by aliens to destroy the human race
Good?	Yes	Yes	Yes	Yes	Never, no, blech!
Ratio to eat relative to other fats?	1/3	1/6	1/6	1/3	#DIV/o!*
Typically Reduce or Increase?	Reduce	Increase	Reduce	Increase	Destroy!

Table 8 Fat Table: The Table Itself Isn't Fat. It's Just Big Boned.

---

* Microsoft Excel humor.

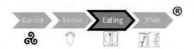

If you hate tables, with their beautiful rows and columns majestically presenting data in a structured manner (sigh), here's a narrative recommendation about how to honor mantra #5. It assumes your only goal is to adopt a healthier diet. More specific goals may require tweaks.

- Omega-3 and monounsaturated fats are good fats. Increase the amounts in your diet.
- Saturated and omega-6 fats are also good fats. You probably get plenty already. If you increase Omega-3 and monounsaturated fats, you may need to reduce saturated and omega-6 fats to keep your calorie consumption in check. Another way to compensate for the calories is to reduce refined carbohydrates.
- Trans fats are bad fats. They are one of the few things I ask you to never, ever eat. Other things on this list include arsenic, hemlock, cyanide, ricin, and Ben & Jerry's Chubby Hubby. The last item has special disposal instructions. If you have any, just send it to me, I am a licensed Chubby Hubby disposal expert.

Make sure the fats you eat are evenly represented from each major category (i.e. saturated, polyunsaturated, and monounsaturated). Also, within the category of polyunsaturated fats, have a one-to-one ratio of omega-3s to omega-6s. But no need to go all OCD about this. If you increase the amount of monounsaturated and omega-3 fats, you're probably OK.

The typical North American diet is one of our top five worst exports to the rest of the world. Among its problems are spates of foods with cheap omega-6 vegetable oils and foods deep fried in saturated or trans fat. These fats crowd out the monounsaturated and omega-3 fats that we should be eating. In case you're wondering, the other exports in the top five are the song "Cotton Eyed Joe," Shake Weights, the TV show *Manimal*, and Ben & Jerry's Chubby Hubby (like the United States' precious domestic oil, we should be hoarding that last one).

For some of you, this information may be more than enough to honor mantra #5 as well as to live long and prosper.

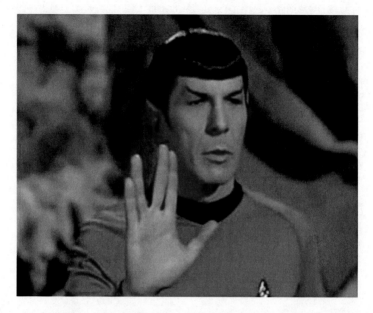

Figure 41 Vulcans are Generally Vegetarians. They Eat Meat When No Other Protein is Available. They Rarely Drink Alcohol. Leave it to Vulcans to Have Karma Sense.[128,129]

Others are masochists and can continue reading to learn specifics about why these fats are good, why you may have been led to believe otherwise, the dangers of the pendulum swinging the other way, and most importantly, how to cut through the incredible misinformation (which I believe is what classy people say when they really mean "utter bullcrap") and manage your intake in a way that makes you healthier, happier, and you guessed it, saves the world.

We'll start with exploring what fat was like before rumors encumbered it. Like my friend, fat was just getting by.

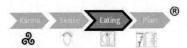

Getting By

The funny thing about rumors is that no matter what they claim, they never change the truth. Here is the truth about fat and why your body needs it:

- It forms a critical part of our nervous system (including our brains) and our endocrine system (including sexy-time). A proper mix of fats in the diet ensures that these two systems are on their best behavior.
- It provides structure to our cell membranes. A balanced mix of the good fats makes sure cell membranes are neither too stiff nor too fluid (those adjectives are *not* related to sexy-time).
- It provides *essential* nutrients. When applied to nutrition, *essential* means nutrients that can only be acquired from the diet or through supplements. This is in contrast to other nutrients which our body can make on its own with ingredients stored in the cupboard. While the body can convert many types of fatty acids into other types of fat, two are considered essential. These are linolenic acid and linoleic acid used to make omega-3 and omega-6 fats. These fatty acids are critical to the nervous system and to manage your body's inflammation response.
- It allows absorption of other essential nutrients, such as the fat-soluble vitamins A, D, E and K. These nutrients are not absorbed by the body unless consumed with fat.
- It provides more energy than any other macronutrients.
- Face it, it improves the flavor of many foods that we eat.

I think you'd agree, fat has a lot going for it. Is it perfect? No. Even before the rumors started, fat had some legitimate issues:

- It provides more energy than any of the macronutrients. You might be thinking, "Hey, didn't you just say that was one of its positive aspects?" Yes, I did. But this means gram-for-gram, fat has a lot of calories (nine calories per gram vs. four calories per gram for protein or carbs). Calorie density is the reason fat can make you fat.

- Favoring one type of fat in the diet over other type makes many of the features listed above disappear. The North American Diet tends to favor saturated and cheap, über-inflammatory omega-6 fats.

- Certain totally awesome fats (e.g., olive oil) are mishandled. They're stored improperly (in bright, warm environments), they're stored for too long, or they're used for high heat cooking. These practices turn them from anti-inflammatory superheroes to inflammatory zeroes.

You can see how, with some clever handling of this information, one could turn a perfectly good friend into a scapegoat.

Scapegoat

It started innocently enough. In the mid-twentieth century, there was a revolution in food production. Technologies and advancements improved automation, fertilizers, feeds, pesticides, irrigation, preservation, packaging, husbandry, flavor, and appearance. According to data from the US Department of Commerce, year-over-year productivity from farm-to-table improved five times from what it had been just a few decades earlier.[130] The bottom line is that delicious, affordable calories became available on an unprecedented scale.

Meanwhile, on the other side of the tracks, well-meaning medical researchers were alarmed by the increase in chronic conditions such as cancer, heart disease, and Type 2 Diabetes. In searching for an answer, they made a correlation between the increased consumption of saturated fat and these medical conditions. The flaws in these studies are beyond the scope of this book but, if you're interested in learning more, I recommend <u>the excellent write-up</u> by Dr. David Katz.[131] Furthermore, *all*

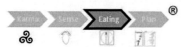

sources of dietary fat were demonized even though the research focused solely on saturated fats.

These findings were picked up quickly by some of the very same consumer goods companies that were the true cause of the problems to begin with (Note: These consumer goods companies are also members of the Tasty-But-Empty-Calorie Cabal. They get around). As a dues-paying member of the HIC, they conspire to motivate consumer behavior in the direction most beneficial to them. Other members of the HIC include the big pharma, medical device, and care delivery companies that fund scientific research in hopes of uncovering new benefits for their products. The research community either has to play along or see its funding dry up. Armed with these "discoveries," the marketers then cajole (really, they're always cajoling) the media to publicize their findings or lose precious advertising dollars. This increased demand makes people sicker. It is the most vicious of cycles.

This version of fat shaming resulted in an avalanche of products responding to the wrong problem, products that were worse than the conditions they were meant to resolve. Unless those conditions were sagging profits for food manufacturers, in which case their products kicked butt. I'm talking about completely unsatisfying fat-free cheese that only makes you ache for something probably worse. Sugar infused fat-free dressing that prevents you from absorbing all of the fat-soluble vitamin goodness in the salad you're eating. And, the Frankenfood that would make any GMO tomato blush—fat-free cookies and pastries. "Food" so odious, it made me stop typing so I could look up what "odious" means. Case in point:

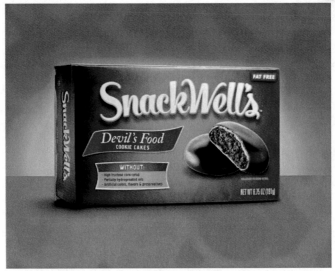

Figure 42 It's not Called Devil's Food for Nothing.[132]

Ingredients: Sugar (1st ingredient, sugar), *Enriched Flour* (2nd ingredient, refined starch), *[Wheat Flour, Niacin, Reduced Iron, Thiamine Mononitrate, (Vitamin B1) Riboflavin (Vitamin B2), Folic Acid], High Fructose Corn Syrup* (3rd ingredient, sugar), *Corn Syrup* (4th ingredient, sugar), *Skim Milk, Cocoa (Processed With Alkali), Glycerin, Emulsifiers [(Adds A Trivial Amount of Fat) Soy Lecithin, Mono - and Diglycerides], Leavening (Baking Soda, Sodium Aluminum Phosphate, Calcium Phosphate), Gelatin,* **Cornstarch** (refined starch)**, Modified Corn Starch** (refined starch), *Chocolate (Adds A Trivial Amount of Fat), Salt, Potassium Sorbate Added to Preserve Freshness,* **Artificial Flavor** (mmmmm, faux flavor).

So we had a scapegoat, fat. We had a response to said scapegoat, fat-free atrocities. And all the chronic conditions that started this brouhaha only got worse. Meanwhile, in defiance of the HIC, an unheard minority was achieving fabulous results with higher fat diets. The Atkins and South Beach plans practically eliminated carbs from the diet, and people who followed them lost weight and watched their heart health improve. On the other side of the tracks (the same side as the aforementioned well-meaning medical researchers), more balanced, high-fat diets that included carbs also received attention for their health benefits. The Mediterranean Diet, rich in omega-3s, monounsaturated oils, and

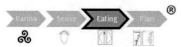

loads of plant-based foods including whole grains, were linked to heart health and longevity.

Where are we in this story (I was getting lost too)? Dietary fat was scapegoated as a major health issue. Removing fat from the diet only worsened the health problem. People who resisted the low-fat trend ended up healthier than those who followed it. Maybe we had it all wrong about fat. Maybe fat is cool. But is fat heroic?

Hero?

Fat is now at the same point in the story as my friend when he joined the cool crowd. And based on how things are playing out, the parallels to that story may continue. The benefits of higher fat diets are becoming common knowledge. Most telling, the 2015 Dietary Guidelines Advisory Committee is beginning to distance itself from erroneous claims linking dietary cholesterol, fat and heart disease.[133] The committee, however, still demonizes saturated fats although the evidence does not support a link to the chronic disease epidemic.[134]

The only people left who still believe the low-fat dogma are the same folks who are miffed that TV executives canceled *Murder She Wrote*. The cool kids now eat their bacon-wrapped-buffalo-chicken-wings at about 200 calories per wing and a full day's calories per serving (but low-carb!). Or they're eating potato chips cooked in olive oil. The same olive oil that is damaged during high heat deep frying. And new Frankenfoods find their way to the grocery store shelves. Food so odious that it made me forget what "odious" means so I had to look it up again. Case in point:

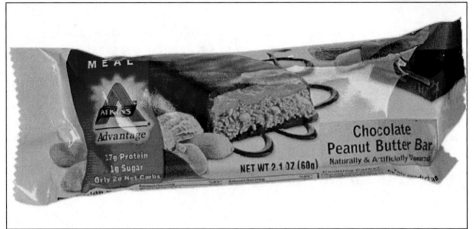

Figure 43 Atkins Advantage Bar - Our Advantage is the Dipotassium Phosphate.[135]

Ingredients: Chocolate Flavored Coating (Polydextrose (gross), Palm Kernel Oil, Whey Protein Isolate, Cocoa Powder (Processed with Alkali), Soy Lecithin, Artificial Flavor (gross), Sucralose (gross), Acesulfame Potassium (gross)), Peanut Butter Flavored Layer (Maltitol (gross), Palm Kernel and Palm Oil, Peanut Butter, Partially Defatted Peanut Flour, Nonfat Dry Milk, Whey Powder, Peanuts, Salt, Soy Lecithin, Anhydrous Milk Fat, Cocoa Powder (Processed with Alkali), Glycerin, Protein Blend (Soy Protein Isolate, Whey Protein Isolate, Sodium Caseinate), Peanuts, Hydrolyzed Gelatin, Water, Polydextrose (still gross), Peanut Butter (Ground, Roasted Peanuts), Cellulose, Natural and Artificial Flavors (gross), Palm Kernel Oil, Olive Oil, Clarified Butter, Soy Lecithin, Guar Gum, Vitamin Mineral Mix (Tricalcium Phosphate, Calcium Carbonate, Magnesium Oxide, Vitamin A Palmitate, Ascorbic Acid (Vitamin C), Sodium Ascorbate, Thiamine Mononitrate (Vitamin B1), Riboflavin (Vitamin B2), Pyridoxine Hydrochloride (Vitamin B6),DL-Alpha Tocopheryl Acetate (Vitamin E), Niacinamide, Biotin, D-Calcium Pantothenate, Zinc Oxide, Folic Acid, Chromium Chelate, Phytonadione (Vitamin K1), Sodium Selenite, Cyanocobalamin (Vitamin B12), Salt, Maltodextrin, Citric Acid, Sucralose (gross), Mono and Diglycerides, Dipotassium Phosphate (gross)).

The list above is more deceptively problematic than the SnackWell's list (and don't get me started on SnackWell's incorrect use of the apostrophe). The length of ingredients alone should give you pause. Words to live by: Avoid eating any packaged foods with more ingredients than there are states in the United States. And the chemical additives! Oy vey! The bar contains loads of vitamins, but they're

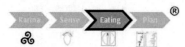

synthetic and your body doesn't absorb synthetic vitamins well. Then there are the sugar alcohols and soy derivatives that are known to give many people belly aches or worse. My fear is that while fat is becoming cool, we're falling into the same trap we were in when it was demonized. It's one extreme or the other. It's all or nothing. If only there were a dogma-free place to guide our nutrition choices. A place that respected individual needs, preference, and goals. Hmmm...

The Karma Sense Eating Plan

The Karma Sense Eating Plan is designed to be inclusive. There are no cool kids. There are no losers. We all exist together in one giant, good karma, "Kumbaya" conclave. So we're going to make this as simple and stress-free as possible. First, the best way to manage your dietary fat is to follow all the plan's mantras. By doing so, you're starting off with a very good mix of nutrients and blocking some of the bad actors we want to avoid. Next be sure to:

Eat More Omega-3 Polyunsaturated Fats

Omega-3s lower your cells viscosity (makes them more supple). By increasing fluidity, your muscle cells become more sensitive to insulin. Having fluid cells also helps the nervous system and the brain communicate more efficiently. Your grandma may have told you fish was brain food. Your grandma was a freaking neuroscientist who could make a kicka$$ salmon casserole. Omega 3s are also critical to the immune system. They are anticoagulant, anti-inflammatory catalysts to blood vessel and respiratory system dilation, and they reduce pain.

Ways to get more omega-3s, ranked from most effective to least effective (but all are worthwhile), include:

- Eat foods that come from the sea. If you're a vegetarian, that's going to mean algae (but fear not, if slimy green stuff is not to your liking, you have other options). If you do eat fish, smallish wild-caught cold water fish are your best source. They are low in contaminants and high in the fat you want. See the Appendix, Food Lists to learn about your options.

- Supplement with fish oil or algae based omega-3 products.
- Eat flax seeds, hemp seeds (dude), walnuts, and chia seeds. And if you have extra chia seeds, you can do this:

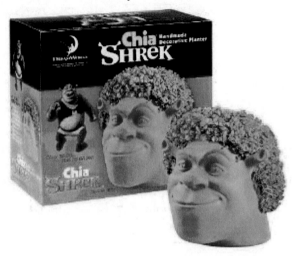

Figure 44 Fat Isn't the Only Misunderstood Ogre.[136]

- Learn about the true fat content of foods that aren't normally associated with omega-3s. There is a misconception that foods like eggs and red meats are nothing but protein and saturated fat. The fact is that an egg's fat is mostly unsaturated. Eggs and beef contain all three major categories of fat. If the animals that produced your eggs and beef were pasture raised and not grain fed, much of their fat content is unsaturated omega-3.

Eat More Monounsaturated Fats

Monounsaturated fats have a similar effect on the cells as omega-3s (i.e., they make the cells gooey - in a good way). They also have a positive effect on blood lipids by decreasing your bad (LDL) cholesterol. Great sources include avocados, almonds, cashews, hazelnuts, macadamias,

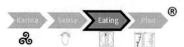

olives, pecans, pistachios, and sesame seeds. Many of these are useful in their pure oil form. Everyone knows about olive oil. If you like living on the edge, mix it up a bit and use macadamia and avocado oils on salads and vegetables. You are a wild child. Sesame oil is quite tasty when cooking Asian style.

Be Mindful of the Omega-6 Polyunsaturated Fats That You Eat

Omega-6s are the yin to the omega-3's immune system yang. Where omega-3s dilate, omega-6s constrict. When omega-3s are "anti," omega-6s are "pro." And, omega-6s can exacerbate pain. Knowing this, you might think you should totally avoid omega-6s but this is not the case. The omega-3s and omega-6s cooperate to support your immune system. When there is an authentic reason for inflammation to occur, you want it to occur. You just don't want chronic inflammation. By keeping your omega fats in balance, these immunity responses are also balanced. Omega-6 fats are plentiful in our diet. Many prepared foods are made with vegetable oils (e.g., soybean) that are high in omega-6 because they are the cheapest (often due to government subsidies, thank you very much). The Karma Sense theory is that by increasing the amount of omega-3s you eat, you achieve balance. But for extra credit, if you remove foods that contain soybean, corn, and other vegetable oils, you'll do yourself (and others) a great service. Because we all want you to be the healthiest you that you can be. We kind of like you (not necessarily "like"-like you, but definitely like you).

Be Mindful of the Saturated Fats that You Eat

Saturated fats caused this whole fat kerfuffle to begin with. Now there's a considerable movement recognizing that saturated fats can actually be beneficial, and associations to various chronic diseases are just as likely to come from conflated unhealthful behaviors (e.g., too many refined carbs, sedentary lifestyle) as from the saturated fat itself. In other words, the cheeseburger may not be the problem. The refined flour bun, potatoes deep fried in highly heated oil, high fructose corn syrup infused tomato sauce (a.k.a., ketchup), and liter of sugar water might be the issue. The fact is, we don't know, but there is likely no harm in controlling saturated fat intake in order to balance saturated with desirable unsaturated fat sources. Furthermore:

- If you eat animal products, you probably consume enough saturated fat. You don't need to increase the amount you eat. If you want to optimize your intake, aim towards animal products grown organically and fed their natural diets (i.e. grass-fed cows, pasture-raised chickens, wild caught fish). This significantly increases omega-3 content and provides a better balance. It also makes for happier animals. *The Karma Sense Eating Plan* does not discriminate by species when it comes to the whole "happy" thing.
- If you avoid animal products, know this, saturated fats in their purest forms are usually solid at room temperature (think butter, schmaltz, and lard). Coconut and palm oils are good sources. Feel free to cook with these tasty, healthful oils. Vegetable shortening and margarine are hydrogenated forms of vegetable oil. They are trans fat Frankenfoods and odious (I remembered this time!). I know the plan is inclusive and everything but it does not include eating chemically saturated fats. Other prohibited activities include looking directly at a total solar eclipse, playing in the middle of traffic, listening to The Starland Vocal Band's "Afternoon Delight" or sharing my Ben & Jerry's Chubby Hubby ice cream (except with my wife. May I sleep in my own bed now?).

Trans Fats - No!

Like cheap vegetable oils, hydrogenation is an awesome technology for stockholders in companies that make up the Tasty-But-Empty-Calorie

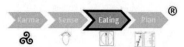

Cabal. It's cheap. It improves the taste of foods that would be inedible without it. And it lasts forever so that foods containing trans fats can survive a nuclear holocaust. The upside is that if the holocaust were to cause an epidemic of Giant Nuclear Monsters, we could feed them Ho-Hos from our strategic junk food stockpile, and they'd all die of chronic diseases.

The best way to avoid trans fats is to check product ingredients. If they contain partially hydrogenated anything, they contain trans fats. Don't rely on the label's nutrition facts. Consumer goods companies paid attention in math class. They figured out how to manipulate serving sizes and FDA regulations so they can say chips containing partially hydrogenated soybean oil have 0% trans fats, as long as you restrict your consumption to one chip. And really, who can eat just one?

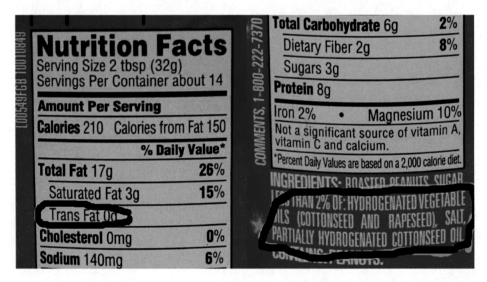

Figure 45 Liar![137]

One more comment about trans fats, and I'll get off my high horse (how the horse got high, I'll never know. Hemp seeds?). Nut butters are a great source of healthy fats. They can also be great sources of trans fats. If you buy nut butters in jars that you don't have to stir, they probably contain a crapload of trans fats. Buy natural nut butters that require stirring. Store them upside down so the oil mixes into the nut goo. After you open and stir, keep them in the refrigerator, and they won't separate again. You can also make your own nut butter. Many supermarkets have the machines in-store so you can do so.

Two Additional Notes on Fats and I'll Give You a Break

Oils can be very volatile. Not "terrible-two" volatile, but pretty unstable. If mishandled, even anti-inflammatory fats can cause inflammation. Be aware of oil's shelf life before you buy. Don't buy oils in massive quantities if you're not going to use them within a few months. If they smell rancid, throw them out. Aim for expeller and cold pressed oils vs. chemically extracted oils. Chemical extraction is a cheap process that makes your oil yucky (which I believe is a technical term for "causes inflammation").

Oils last longer when you store them in the refrigerator. It's a bit of a pain because some solidify at colder temperatures, but you can loosen them up by running the bottle under warm water for a few minutes.

When cooking with oil make sure you use one that is right for the temperature required. Olive oil, for example, has a low smoke point which means it burns when exposed to high heat. Burned oil is inflammatory oil. Check the labels and cook with healthy high heat oils. A small contingent of The Militia will tell you never to cook with fats, especially at high heat. C'mon?!? That's crazy talk! They obviously never experienced the joy of roasted broccoli (or the occasional french fry).

So, before moving on to special considerations and key points, we probably should predict what will become of fat. Will fat's story mirror that of my friend who was ultimately eaten by a Giant Nuclear Monster? I really don't know. But if a Giant Nuclear Monster eats fat using Karma Sense, Tokyo doesn't stand a chance.

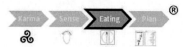

Special Considerations

It's time to explore how people with different goals should adjust the mantra of Eat Good Fats Daily and Balance a Variety of Good Fats.

Lose Weight

Follow the guidelines for balancing fats described in this mantra. Be especially careful with overall fat intake because of the high number of calories. If you follow the other mantras, especially mantra #3, Eat Whole Food Carbohydrates After Vigorous Exercise, you should have no problem losing weight. If you find you're not losing as much as you want, aim for leaner versions of protein and lessen the amount of oil used to prepare your meals.

Maintain Weight but Eat Healthier

Follow the guidelines of good fat balance as described in this mantra. Try not to include high-fat and high-carb meals in the same day. But what's the problem with a little gnocchi with pesto every once in a while?

Gain Weight in the Form of Muscle

Follow the guidelines of good fat balance as described in the mantra.

Key Points

1. Fat is another misunderstood macronutrient. Your goal is to focus on getting the right mix of different fats instead of restricting or eliminating fats.
2. There are three major categories of fats. They are saturated, monounsaturated, and polyunsaturated fats. Aim to get a good mix of each.

3. Of the polyunsaturated fats, there are two essential ones that you must eat. They are omega-3 and omega-6 polyunsaturated fats. Aim to eat a balanced mix.

4. Do not eat foods that contain trans fats. Ever. I really mean it.

5. The typical diet in the developed world contains sufficient saturated fats and omega-6 polyunsaturated fats. Try to increase your intake of monounsaturated and omega-3 fats, and reduce your intake of saturated and omega-6 polyunsaturated fats.

6. Managing fat intake may require reading the ingredient and nutrition fact labels on packaged foods.

7. Store oils properly and use them for the cooking job for which they are intended. Most monounsaturated oils are not good for high heat cooking.

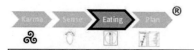

Karma Sense in the Wild

I met Ryan several years ago at a technology entrepreneur networking event back when I was recruiting sales people and engineers for my startup. We had a lot in common. We went to the same university at about the same time. We both majored in computer science. And we attended the networking event for the same reason. We were trying to find traction for some bleeding edge ideas we had. One final similarity is that we track our biomarkers using various tools so we can analyze our health. However, our motivations are very different. I do it because I have an unnatural, irrational, and insatiable curiosity about health. Ryan's motivation is an internal ticking time bomb.

I learned about this ticking time bomb at a more recent networking event. Ryan had heard about my new career as an Integrative Health Coach and wanted to talk to me about some concerns he had. Apparently the males in his family have a history of early heart disease, and several had heart attacks before turning age 60.

To Ryan's credit, he leads a healthy lifestyle. He doesn't let stress get to him, he exercises, and he eats well. As a self-declared member of the "quantitative self" movement, he knows his numbers, and his cholesterol was troubling him. When first tested, Ryan's total cholesterol was borderline high (over 200 mg/dl). In response to this test, he made some lifestyle changes, and over time his total cholesterol dropped to well within the healthy range. The bad news was that his HDL, the good cholesterol, fell significantly below where his doctor and conventional wisdom wants to see it (less than 35 mg/dl).

I asked Ryan about his lifestyle changes and how he achieved his radical reduction. Apparently, he adopted a very low-fat diet based on what he read by Dr. Dean Ornish. As previously noted, Dr. Ornish's low-fat philosophy is currently under question, but it works for many and it worked for Ryan. Ryan reviewed his current diet with me and it's quite wholesome. It consists mostly of oatmeal, vegetables and fruits. For protein he primarily eats chicken but mixes it up with a little fish. Red meat is a rare treat. He eats pasta about twice a week and hardly ever touches bread, rice, or potatoes.

I shared some resources on the latest research and thinking on the role of fat in the diet and specifically on ways to increase one's HDL. As a result of that discussion, Ryan began supplementing regularly with fish oil (omega-3s). He also made a small serving of mixed nuts (omega-3, omega-6, and monounsaturated fats) part of his daily routine. Before he made these additions, Ryan's fat intake was low, but highly slanted towards saturated fats. By making these changes to his diet he ensured that he was Eating Good Fats Daily and Balancing a Variety of Good Fats.

I checked in with Ryan a couple months later because I knew he intended to have his lipids checked soon after we talked. In that time his HDL had increased 10%. He still has a way to go, and if he remains committed to raising his HDL, there are other changes I'd suggest. For now, we'll watch and wait.

Plan

Playing With *The Karma Sense Eating Plan*

Executive Summary

If ever you wake up in the middle of the night with an exciting idea; an idea with the expansive goal of helping people be healthier, be happier, and, oh yeah, save the world; an idea that achieves these goals in a way that is flexible, inclusive and tolerant; be prepared. Be prepared for your labor of love to be all consuming. Be prepared for second-guessing and self-doubt. Be prepared for the injuries from banging your head against the wall as you try to find an approachable way to articulate your thoughts. And know that, if your idea survives all that, the real challenge is yet to come.

Now the hard work begins. The description of the *Plan* component has to honor all this modularity, flexibility, and individuality, but still help you reach your end goal. Everyone wants to be healthier, happier, and make the world a better place, and what that looks like to each person is different. So my approach to tie all this together is similar to what you get with a Lego set. You buy it to build the pirate ship.

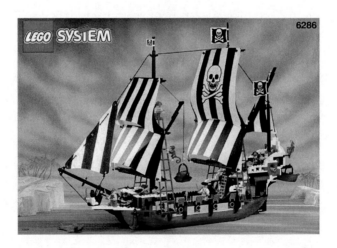

Figure 46 Avast Matey! Thar's Nuttin but Empty Chubby Hubby Containers on This Here Island.[138]

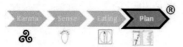

But sooner or later, you're pulling off the monkey's head and making it stick out of one of the cannons, and you're decapitating a pirate and shoving his torso neck first into the shark's mouth. You're personalizing the scene. Next thing you know, you rearrange the blocks to turn the pirate ship into a pirate rocket ship.

This chapter describes how to build a pirate ship. It also tells you what to consider when building *your* pirate ship. And it does so without ever having to worry about stepping on those darn bricks when you're walking around barefoot. Note that this chapter simply describes the process. The Appendix includes tools and references to help you develop all aspects of your plan in a very structured way.

But before digging deeper, I have to set some expectations.

Disclaimers

Disclaimer 1 - I am Still Not a Doctor.

Among other subjects, this plan is concerned with your health. The conventional medical community is very protective of this domain. The initial discussion of the Karma and Sense components explore aspects of health that conventional medicine is only just beginning to tackle. It's the mind-over-matter part. Even mantra #1 of the Eating component, Eat Slowly and Stop Before You're Full, is advice you're unlikely to get from a physician. However, as soon as I start talking about what you eat, I begin walking the fine line between good old common sense (more like great new Karma Sense) and medical advice. Do not construe any aspect described in this plan as a prescription for disease treatment or as medical advice. If you have any questions about how the plan affects health, please consult someone on your medical health care team.

Disclaimer 2 - This Chapter Demonstrates My Attention Deficit Issues Even More Than its Predecessors

In the introductory Overview chapter, I describe my struggle over using the label "Plan" to identify the last component. At first, creating a plan around a set of common sense and healthy behaviors you can adopt or ignore at your own pace seemed like a fool's errand. Then I realized I was just the fool for the job, and I've grown accustomed to the term. While the plan is loosey-goosey, it can be structured into a sort-of-blueprint for better health that achieves very specific results. This chapter covers the many different considerations you should explore if you have the motivation and knowledge to assemble a structured plan by yourself. To cover everything, I'm forced to skip across a variety of subjects. The resulting text may lack some of the coherence you've come to expect. (Editor's Note: Coherence? Is that what you call it?). As I jump around the different subjects, please be patient, as there will be some attempt to tie it all together in the end.

Disclaimer 3 - This Chapter Primarily Discusses Customization of the Eating Component. This Does not Minimize the Importance of the Karma and Sense Components.

Karma, gratitude, and mindfulness (a.k.a., doing nothing) are essential to the plan. However, the plan defers to your own definition of good deeds, gratitude, and doing nothing because your good feelings about the outcomes drive these actions.

The guidelines for eating, however, depend more on the science of good nutrition. They are driven by the less flexible laws of physics, chemistry, and biology. Therefore, the customizations discussed below mostly plug away at the Eating component. Please do not assume that this focus on Eating minimizes the importance of Karma and Sense. You maximize

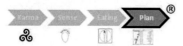

opportunities for happiness and world-saving when you implement all components.

Wow, these disclaimers are the most serious things I've written since the time I misbehaved in school and had to do a hundred word essay on why I shouldn't call a teacher a "stinky poopy head." Even after I finished the essay, my organic chemistry professor never really forgave me for that slight. And speaking of forgiveness, forgive me the indulgence of providing a brief overview of *The Karma Sense Eating Plan*. Think of it as the instruction sheet they shove in your box of Legos.

The Karma Sense Eating Plan Overview

People have different learning styles. So I offer this overview in three formats.

Text Description

The Karma Sense Eating Plan mixes the science of behavior change, gratitude, and nutrition, and sprinkles it liberally with some faith in your fellow humans. Its goal is to support your health, happiness, and the greater good. The entire process flows like this:

Perform a good deed that is not part of your current routine. The more the good deed is associated with food, the better. The closer the good deed is performed to your mealtime, the better. Do something *you* consider to be good. Don't worry about someone else's definition. In the end, everyone's combined goodness will even out. It's the crowd-sourced way to save the world.

- Before eating all meals, stop to reflect on:
    - Your good deeds
    - Something good someone did for you that is worthy of your appreciation (reverse karma)
    - The effort that went into preparing your food
- When eating, honor the following mantras:

- o Eat Slowly and Stop Before You're Full
- o Eat Protein in Every Meal
- o Eat More Vegetables and Fruits
- o Eat Whole Food Carbohydrates After Vigorous Exercise
- o Eat Good Fats Daily and Balance a Variety of Good Fats

Visual Description

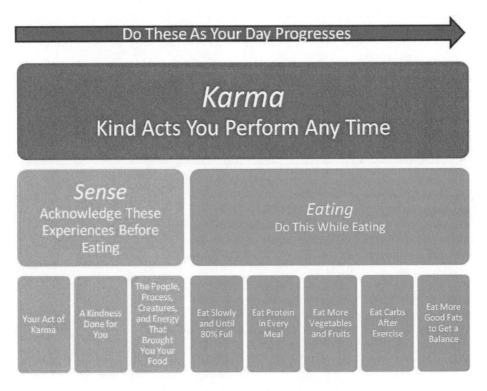

Figure 47 Eleven Rectangles of Karma Sense Eating.[139]

Description in Verse

Sung to the Tune of "50 Ways to Leave Your Lover" (with apologies to Paul Simon)[140]

"The problem's all inside your head,"
I say to thee.

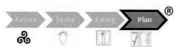

"There's many ways for
You to become healthy.
And in the process
You can also be happy.
There's many nifty ways
To do the Karma."

I say, "I know you'd really
Like to save the world."
Your skepticism shows
Your mouth becomes all curled.
But I'll repeat myself
As this plan is
Unfurled.
"There's many nifty ways
To do the Karma."

There's Do a Good Deed, Reed.
Shake up your Habit, Rabbit. *
Eat Less Quick, Mick.
Eat More Protein, Jean.
Fill up on Plants, Lance.
Time your Carbs, Barb.
Balance your Fat, Pat.
See what I mean?

Sorry. I got carried away with the name rhyming thing and the meter fell out of step with the original song at the end. But, it remains true to *The Karma Sense Eating Plan*. And in case you're wondering, I am available for weddings, bar mitzvahs, and bachelorette parties.

---

* The main character from the movie *Eight Mile*. If great literature is more your thing, feel free to replace with Rabbit from *Winnie the Pooh* (foreshadowing). Or, if you're a grown-up, Babbitt from Sinclair Lewis' *Babbitt*. The important thing here is that it's not easy to find names that rhyme with "habit."

Now that you're reacquainted with the different blocks in the Lego set, let's figure out what you want to make.

What Do I Need to Know to Make a Karma Sense Plan?

You can go through a series of thought exercises to maximize your plan's chance of success. The exercises help you look at the big picture of your health and happiness before working out the details of a plan. By linking the details back to the big picture, you always remember why you're engaged in this process. It's an activity that helps you maintain motivation. <u>Research</u> shows that we humans are more likely to succeed at positive behavior change when that change is aligned to what we view as important.[141] Here is a visual image of the process.

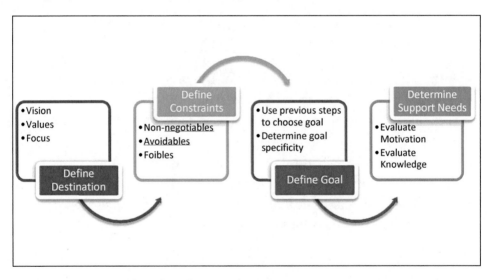

Figure 48 What You Should Know to Develop Your Karma Se nse Eating Plan[142]

Your Destination

Before making *any* changes in the name of better health and happiness, figure out why you want to make these changes in the first place. I find this to be a valuable exercise with everything I do. (e.g., Why am I waking up in the morning? Why am I going to work? Why do I want to

---

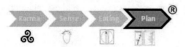

smack Nelson in accounting? Why didn't I smack Nelson in accounting? (karma))

If you're considering adopting the plan, it's probably for at least one of the following reasons:

1. You're bored.
2. You're easily open to suggestion.
3. Someone else is making you (e.g., you're in a hostage situation).
4. You want to achieve something.

Let's explore that last one. To achieve stuff it helps to have a clear understanding of what that "thing" is. Yogi Berra encapsulated this idea best with these words of wisdom:

"If you don't know where you're going, you might not get there." [143]

Mr. Berra is well-known for his head-scratchers. In this sense, he and I are very similar. But he nailed this one. The biggest reason people fail to reach their goals is because they don't really understand the goals. They may know they want to lose weight, but they don't truly understand why it's important to them. Or perhaps they know they want someday to run around with their children and grandchildren, but they don't know what changes to make to ensure they can. Maybe climbing Mt. Everest is on their bucket list, and on that list it will remain because they have no idea how to turn a dream into reality.

A great place to start is to develop a vivid understanding of vision, values, and focus. There are people whose professional careers concentrate on helping others gain that understanding. I know because I am one (contact me ☺).

Although I obviously believe there is great value in working with a professional health coach to find your "thing," it's not a requirement. In the Appendix Plan Tools, I give some lightning round questions you can ask yourself to navigate from the bird's eye view of where you want your health to be to the bug's eye level of detail (e.g., "What exactly does that look like?"). Here's a sample of the questions:

Vision

- When you think about your best future, how far ahead do you look (e.g., five years, ten years, six months)?
- In that future, how will you feel mentally and physically?
- What will you be doing? Answer this one as completely as possible and address who, what, where, when, and how (e.g., who are you with?).

Values

- What matters most to you in life?
- What is it about your vision that stands out as a reflection of what matters to you?
- What strengths do you have that will help you achieve your vision?
- What improvements do you feel you need to make to achieve your vision?

Focus

While thinking about the improvements you need to make, consider:

- Which ones seem most important?
- Which ones seem most difficult to achieve?
- Which are achievable within the time frame of your vision?
- Which changes are you most confident about making now?
- How could you describe these changes so they become discrete actions that drive better health and happiness?

By developing the complete picture of what you want for the healthy, happy version of you, you end up with everything you need to map out

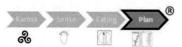

the rest of your course. This vision is useful to refer back to when you feel your willpower waning. But don't fret if a thought exercise like the one above doesn't work for you. As you progress through the planning process, we've got you covered.

Now that you're comfortable with your new definition of health and happiness, the next considerations are your constraints.

Constraints

Knowing where you want to go is a great start. Next take a realistic look at your non-negotiables, desired avoidables, and plain old foibles. Any plan that refuses to accept who you are may make you healthier, but it won't make you happier. And if you're not happy, you're not going to stick to it. Worst of all, unhappy people are generally pretty bad at saving the world.

Take some time to consider these aspects before diving into the Karma Sense pool. Here are some questions to ask.

Non-negotiables

Non-negotiables are things you either won't do or won't give up.

- What foods will you never eat because they violate some value or because the thought of them ties your stomach in a knot?
- What foods must be included in your diet because the thought of never eating them makes you sad, lonely, scared, or violent?
- What aspects of your life complicate your eating habits (e.g., travel, shift work, traditional family meals, or living next door to Five Guys)?

As an example, my non-negotiables are that I won't totally give up ice cream, beer, or wine. I won't eat most organs (because they're gross), and I won't eat turkey (because these days they're mostly genetically engineered monsters and not that delicious). I travel a lot for work. And I live across the street from a bar with a great beer selection.

Avoidables

Avoidables are similar to non-negotiables but you're not as locked in to them. They're a little more challenging to uncover.

- What foods present a value conflict (e.g., you like a specific food, but it violates one of your principles)?
- What foods would you like to eat more often but don't due to some limitation in your environment (e.g., you want to eat more broccoli but you haven't found a preparation that you like)?
- What foods do you think you should eat less often or believe you can reduce the amount you consume, but just haven't done so yet?
- What situations do you typically face that challenge your discipline or self-control (e.g., you can't walk past a coffee shop without buying a giant coffee milkshake, and there's a coffee shop on every corner)?

My avoidables are pork, which I love in many forms but hate the way the brilliant creatures providing my pancetta are treated. I'd like to cut back my animal consumption in general but haven't found a way that easily jives with my fitness goals and schedule. I can usually say no to french fries but do like them when they're well made or when I have an occasional craving. And, between the hours of 8:30 pm and 10:30 pm, it is very difficult for me to decline an offer of easily accessible ice cream.

Foibles

Foibles are your totally weird beliefs or habits that impact how and what you eat, like being grossed out when one of the foods on your plate touches other foods. Or having to remove all the brown M&Ms before eating any. Whatever it is, let your freak flag fly!

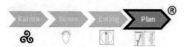

I don't have any foibles. Everything I do is normal. So I can offer no personal examples. Now excuse me while I deconstruct my Ho-Ho (which I believe is what people who aren't from the Northeastern US call "Yodels").

In the end, this collection of constraints may have no effect on your plan's implementation at all. But you don't want to develop a plan only to discover it was doomed to fail from the start because you didn't include constraints in your thought process.

As a result of this exercise, you now have a complete inventory of everything that is important in your life. It should include your thoughts on:

- How active and rested you want to be.
- How you want to nourish your body and your soul.
- Who the people are that matter to you.
- Where you want to be physically and mentally.
- How you want to spend your time.
- Any themes that tie all these together

No matter how far you got in this exercise, you're at the point where you can lay out your plan and can tie it to your goal.

Goal

You're now ready to define your Karma Sense Eating goal. The goal's specificity directly relates to how much progress you made in the previous exercises. For the sake of discussion, we'll assume three levels of specificity. And because I'm such a creative fellow, I'll call them *low*, *medium* and, *high*.

Low Specificity

If you want to proceed with *The Karma Sense Eating Plan* even though your vision is not well developed, you'll probably end up with a low specificity goal. These tend to be Big Hairy Audacious Goals (BHAGs) such as "I want to be healthier, happier, and, oh yeah, save the world." The advantage of a BHAG is that you have a lot more flexibility with implementation. The disadvantage is that it's difficult to observe your progress. If you're a laid-back, mellow, non-striving sort of cat, you may not need to see improvement. On the other hand, if you're someone who is motivated by demonstrable progress, you need the full vision and more specificity or, as Yogi said, you might not get there. In the end, it's up to you. Keep in mind that professional support is available when you're ready. Another resource comes from cranking up your good karma deeds, which expands your friendship circle and provides you a posse of people to give support (you're in the Zone of Trust and Support). That's not necessarily why you're doing good karma deeds. It's just a side benefit.

Medium Specificity

Medium specificity goals are similar to those in the Special Considerations sections of each mantra's chapter. These include, but are not limited to:

- Lose weight
- Maintain weight but be healthier
- Gain weight in the form of muscle

To these, we can add others not tied directly to the Eating component. Examples include:

- Manage stress
- Improve your mindset. Be more optimistic.
- Feel as if you're making a meaningful contribution

The plan can help achieve all these goals. Initially, adopt the components and mantras that are most relevant to you. Like the BHAG, you have flexibility. Unlike the BHAG, you'll find it easier to measure progress.

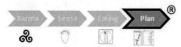

You still may run into motivation traps. How do you know you've lost enough weight or that you're sufficiently happy? There's nothing wrong with not having the answer. If you're comfortable, to quote Abe Lincoln, "Party on, dude!"

High Specificity

With high specificity goals, you know exactly what you want to do and when you want to achieve it. If we look at situations we discussed when exploring Vision, Values, and Focus, these could be:

- *I want to lose weight.* Specifically I want to change my body composition so that my body fat percentage is 15%, and I want to do it by my high school reunion next summer.
- *I want to run around with my children and grandchildren.* I don't usually have much energy, I am not very active, and my vital signs indicate I'm at risk of heart disease. I need to revitalize my energy levels and heart health so I can become more active and be around when my children have children.
- *I want to climb Mt. Everest within the next five years so I can cross that off my bucket list.* This means I need to become leaner and stronger so my arms can support my body weight and I can begin training for the climb.

The plan is perfect for high specificity goals. These goals are very motivating. They can easily translate into specific measurable actions. Also, you can see a direct line to the goal (15% body fat) and the vision (look hot at my high school reunion.) High specificity goals don't allow much flexibility. They require expertise that many people don't have. They're also difficult for people to manage on their own because they require a level of objectivity that's hard to have about oneself. This is a long way for me to say that these goals often require professional support.

Regardless of which level of specificity you've landed upon, you're now ready to build.

Build Your Plan

To form your plan, there are a few more questions to answer.

Do I Need Help and, If So, From Whom?

The answer is, of course, "It depends." Fortunately there are a finite number of variables and outcomes that drive the decision. Think about the goal you settled upon when devising your plan inputs. Now ask these two questions:

- How motivated am I?
- How knowledgeable am I about what it takes to accomplish this?

Depending on the answer, you may want help from one of the following:

- Nobody - You're a loner. A rebel.

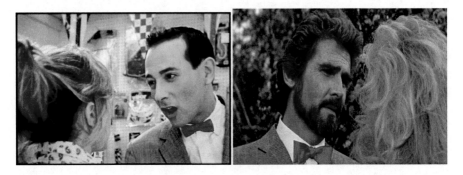

Figure 49 We Know You Are, Dotties, But What Are We?[144,145]

- Nutrition Coach - Someone who appreciates your goals and constraints and can teach you how to maneuver.
- Health Coach - Someone who keeps you motivated but provides you the autonomy and space you need to drive your plan on your own.

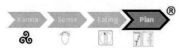

I could explain how to mix and match these in words. But why do that when I can introduce a table?

How High Is Your...		Motivation	
		Low	High
Knowledge	Low	Health Coach	Nutrition Coach
	High	Health Coach	Wild Card

Table 9 What Kind of Support Should You Get?

Beautiful, isn't it? By the way, I deny the rumor that it was once said to me, "Is that a banana in your pocket, or did you just create a table?"

If you decide you want support, your work on the Plan component may be done for now. Identify the coach and move forward with this newfound partner. I hope you consider me. It would be productive and fun.

If you don't know how to look for help, for example, you know Davey H is a coach but you also know a little too much about him at this point and feel he's a bad fit. I'm still happy to help you find the support you need. I have the pleasure of knowing some of the best in the industry and am happy to point you in the right direction. You've been introduced to some of them in this book.

If you don't want support or are still unsure, you have another question to consider.

Which Components and Mantras Are Best Suited to Your Goals?

The Karma Sense Eating Plan is designed so you can adopt it all at once, Big Bang style or implement it in pieces. Which you choose depends on how well you know yourself.

If you are very disciplined, motivated, and open to change, by all means go Big Bang. Otherwise, you should look at each component and mantra closely and prioritize the ones that seem most important, most effective, most likely to bring about the desired change, and easiest to adopt. You should examine these variables in light of the vision, values, focus, and goals you developed.

Keep in mind that this plan is created by and belongs to you. At no time are you obligated to implement the entire plan to reap the benefit. There is a great deal of flexibility in how to comply with the components and mantras. *The Karma Sense Eating Plan* is an open source strategy for optimal health, happiness, and world saving. This means you decide how you participate. I'm only here to help. You can adopt it all or you can select the parts that work for you. But the more you adopt, the more likely you'll reach your goal. That's why I think we can all agree that in many respects, *The Karma Sense Eating Plan* is a lot like...

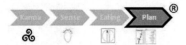

The Mighty Morphin Power Rangers

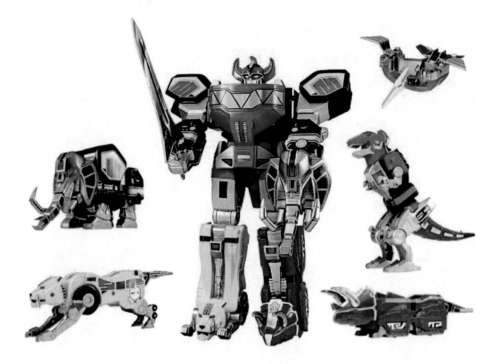

Figure 50 A Giant Nuclear Monster is Attacking Tokyo! It's Morphin Time![146]

If you don't agree, you probably don't know enough about the Mighty Morphin Power Rangers. Lucky for you, this plan can increase your Power Rangers knowledge too.

The *Mighty Morphin Power Rangers* is a TV show and merchandising extravaganza aimed at the attention deficit-prone (I am the target audience). It combines dinosaurs, robots, aliens, monsters, martial arts, loud noises, and bright colors into a panoply of splendor and commercialism (I'm sure you're starting to see the parallels to *The Karma Sense Eating Plan*). Its heroes consist of teenagers of every sex, race, and strata (like the plan, they're inclusive!). They initially fight their enemies in hand-to-hand combat, occasionally supplemented by knife, sword, or stick. If the battle escalates they engage their armored-robotic-extinct-animal-vehicles (a.k.a., Zords) to participate in the fight. And if that doesn't work, their Zords link together and transform into a giant amalgamated robot (Megazord, of course) that never loses. You may ask, "Why not cut to the chase and go right to the Megazord to begin with?" Well, duh, it is Power Rangers creed never to escalate a battle until their opponent does. The Power Rangers may be a cheap and cynical vehicle for selling toys and t-shirts, but they do have standards.

If you want to see the whole ridiculously stupid-awesome scene play out, you can view this 1:45 minute <u>video</u>.[147] But I warn you. I'm not responsible for the diminished IQ points if you watch it.

Speaking of points, I do have a relevant Mighty Morphin Power Ranger point to make. The components and mantras of *The Karma Sense Eating Plan* are like the Power Rangers' Zords. Individually they go a long way in fighting the good fight for better health and happiness. But if you truly want to save the world, combine them all.

To assist in this endeavor, we'll quickly examine how the components interrelate and the implications of adopting them in isolation.

Karma

To execute on the Karma component, you need to perform a good deed that is not part of your normal routine. Making this a habit works wonders in making you happy. It's also your contribution to saving the world. In general, happy people are healthier than unhappy people. But it's difficult for most of us to see the connection between how happy we are and how healthy we are. If I were you, I'd absolutely include the Karma component, the regular performance of some new good deed, in your initial implementation. Fortunately for you, I'm not you. Otherwise, you'd be responsible for this mess.

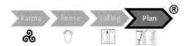

Sense

When you implement the Sense component, you're tying your good deed to how you eat. Introducing this new step into your eating process helps you develop better eating habits for the long term. And the way I ask you to do this also makes you happier. To execute the Sense component, reflect upon the following just before beginning a meal:

- Your good deed and the effect it had on others.
- A kindness performed for your benefit by someone (who could be you) and how you plan to express your gratitude.
- The effort that went into any and all aspects of creating your meal.

On the surface, this seems very easy to do but this is a lot of change to take on. Unless you can develop new habits easily, I recommend you defer implementation of this component until the Karma component is an ingrained habit.

If however, saving the world is not on your agenda, you could adopt the Sense component simply by including the second and third reflections in your pre-meal ritual. Doing these for a sustained period will promote your future happiness.

Eating

The *Eating* component is designed so all five mantras play nicely with each other. By adopting all of them, you build a foundation for good nutrition that will last a lifetime. If you make all five mantras an ingrained habit, you will crowd out the foods that throw your nutrition out of whack. For most of us, adopting all five at once is very difficult. Here's some advice on how to decide and prioritize.

Mantra #1 - Eat Slowly and Stop Before You're Full

This mantra is another aspect that can provide benefit when adopted in isolation without following any other part of the plan. There is no downside to adopting this one while ignoring the rest.

Mantra #2 - Eat Protein in Every Meal

By including more protein in your diet, you should feel fuller sooner and for longer. However, if you do this without adopting mantras #3 and #5, you risk running afoul of some of the overall benefits. For example, mantra #2's description talks about some real issues with excessive protein intake. The vitamins, minerals, and phytonutrients in vegetables and fruits help prevent those negative effects. Meanwhile, whether you are a meat eater or vegetarian, your fat balance can get out of whack unless you deliberately eat the balance of various good fats discussed in mantra #5.

Mantra #3 - Eat More Vegetables and Fruits

There is no downside to adopting this mantra in isolation. Of the mantras that involve specific foods (mantras #2 through #5), it may be the hardest to follow because of people's aversion towards vegetables (and, to a lesser extent, fruits). It's well known that the typical North American diet includes too few vegetables and fruits.[148] The description of mantra #3 includes loads of suggestions on how to work around these difficulties.

Mantra #4 - Eat Whole Food Carbohydrates After Vigorous Exercise

Like mantra #3, this can stand on its own. There is no downside to focusing on whole food sources of carbohydrates and linking them to physical activity. If you're very active, you likely will want to eat carbohydrates more often.

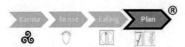

Mantra #5 - Eat Good Fats Daily and Balance a Variety of Good Fats

The key to implementing this mantra's standalone version is to understand your current diet very well. From there, add good fats where your balance is out of whack. Next consider the source of those fats. If you follow the typical North American diet with high saturated and omega-6 polyunsaturated fats, add more monounsaturated and omega-3 polyunsaturated fats to your diet. You can do this with foods or supplements (e.g., pills). I prefer you do this with real food. Either way, you're increasing your calorie count and, unless you make adjustments elsewhere in your diet, you're going to gain weight, most likely as body fat.

So, your honor, I rest my case for the plan's Megazord-i-ness. And like those Mighty Morphin Power Rangers, dedicated to saving the world, you can save the world and your health and happiness as long as you select your implementation plan wisely.

Let's look at a wise implementation plan.

An Example - Choose Foods That Swim, Kim

Kimberly is a gymnast, the Pink Power Ranger, and the master of the Pterodactyl Zord. She needs to maintain her energy and strength so she can perform on the mat and the battlefield. She is particularly concerned about her bone health as she ages because women in her family have a history of osteoporosis. Kimberly likes meat but has some moral issues with consuming animal products. These issues relate partially to the treatment of animals and partially to her belief that, after spending so much time protecting earth from evil monsters, it would be a shame to cause its destruction by encouraging more livestock to consume resources and poop and fart all over the planet. Kimberly is naturally disciplined. Otherwise she wouldn't succeed as a gymnast or as a Power Ranger. However, her busy schedule makes it very difficult to instill change. Kimberly already does quite a bit to save the world but feels she could show more gratitude towards others. How can she reconcile all this and still have Karma Sense?

Kimberly can honor her inner pterodactyl by adopting a diet similar to her Zord's. Pterodactyls primarily ate marine life. By getting most of her protein from wild-caught fish and plant sources, she can honor her moral concerns without going total vegetarian. Many fish are high in calcium as well as omega-3 fats. By combining a shift to fish and plant-based proteins with an increased intake of vegetables, she'll optimize her bone health. Due to the physical stress gymnastics and monster-fighting puts on Kimberly's body, she needs to be sure to get enough carbohydrates. Since she is active, carb timing is less of a concern. Kimberly wants to demonstrate more gratitude and decided to overtly thank the food service employees in her high school cafeteria.

With Kimberly's story, we can create an initial implementation plan. Kimberly decides she can probably take on three new habits at a time. She chooses to do the following every day:

1. Eat one serving of fish or plant-based protein in every meal (mantra #2 with some residual effect from mantra #5).
2. Eat two servings of vegetables at every meal and one serving of fruit twice a day (mantra #3).
3. Thank a high school cafeteria worker every day and complete a positive comment card once a month.

Kimberly understands the rule of thumb that it takes twenty-one days to adopt a new habit. Because her health coach-hero is fond of tables, she creates three tables that look like this (one table for each week):

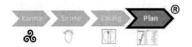

Habit	Su	Mo	Tu	We	Th	Fr	Sa
1 Serving of fish/plant protein for breakfast							
2 Servings of vegetables for breakfast							
1 Serving of fish/plant protein for lunch							
2 Servings of vegetables for lunch							
1 Serving of fish/plant protein for dinner							
2 Servings of vegetables for dinner							
2 Servings of fruit per day							
Thank a high school cafeteria worker	■						■

Table 10 Kimberley's Karma Sense Compliance Tracker

If I was Kimberley, and clearly I am not because pink is not my color, I may structure the table differently. However, this one works for Kimberley. She plans on putting a "✓" in the cell of the table every time she completes the action. You may notice that she did not include the comment card in her table. Since that occurs monthly, she'll just mark a reminder on her calendar app. Also, she blocked out her act of karma on Saturday and Sunday because the school cafeteria is closed on those days.

When Kimberly reaches consistent 90% compliance (to be discussed next) with her new habits, she'll include additional aspects of the plan in her life. She's considering completing support of mantra #5 and adding mantra #1 if she can figure out how to not feel rushed whenever aliens hatch a plot to kidnap the Power Rangers' robot pal, Alpha 5.

And there you have a real life Karma Sense implementation for a fictional character.

But what about this thing called compliance?

Compliance

You would never know it based on what you've read so far, but I'm not delusional. I recognize that expecting 100% conformance to the plan's components and mantras is unreasonable, unrealistic, unexciting, and unbecoming of a cool, fun, fancy-free person such as you. And, it totally goes against good Karma Sense, which begs the question, what is compliance and how do you manage it?

Compliance - What It Is

For something as fungible as this plan, defining and tracking compliance may seem like an exercise in futility. Well, I'm always up for a little exercise. By creating a plan like Kimberly's, we now have something we can follow or ignore. There are two ways to ignore your plan:

- An opportunity arises to invoke one of the habits you plan to adopt, and you don't. In Kimberly's case, this might be forgetting to thank the cafeteria worker at Thursday lunch because she's worried that Zordon, the Power Rangers' mentor, disapproves of her riding her Zord to go to the mall.
- You choose to eat food that's not supported by the plan. For me, that's when I indulge in a little Ben & Jerry's Chubby Hubby and a pint of beer (this is how hubby gets chubby).

Compliance - Managing It

The first thing to keep in mind about *Compliance* is that its counterpart, *N*oncompliance is just as critical. When you choose to be noncompliant, you're not defying the plan. You're identifying times to employ the habits you're developing, and opting not to do so at the time. You're being mind-FUL. There are no good or bad reasons for choosing noncompliance. For the Eating component's mantras, it is just as important to plan for noncompliance as it is to plan for compliance. Here's why:

- As your body adapts to your new super healthy lifestyle, it starts to take the new habits for granted. For example, if you've adopted aspects of the plan to lose weight, over time, your body begins to accommodate to the way you're feeding it. And your weight loss may stall. By throwing your body a curve (Shake It

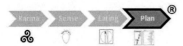

Up!), you can prevent a plateau. Follow this link or footnote to review a <u>study</u> that demonstrates one of the ways this phenomenon manifests itself.[149]

- If you're avoiding certain foods that you normally crave, you feel deprived at times. Every day you go without this food increases the pressure of that craving. If you know in advance that you have the opportunity to eat the food, you relieve the pressure. This too is backed up by <u>research</u>.[150]

- Because I promised you (repeatedly) that the plan was inclusive and is not about taking things away from you, and I keep my promises.

The bottom line is that noncompliance is Karma Science and Karma Sense. Many diet and nutrition experts bristle at the term "noncompliance." Instead, they use the word "refeed." Refeed is a perfectly good name for what you're doing in a plan that focuses solely on nutrition and health. But a plan that focuses on your happiness and enables you to save the world has to go beyond just feeding. Besides, we're grown-ups here (well you people are, I'm more of a man-child). We don't need to sugar-coat things (except on refeed days).

The next thing to consider about compliance is how we measure it. I suggest using a flat percentage. For example, Kimberly's plan calls for 90% compliance. If she is successful during the twenty-one day period, the tables she created for each week would have at least 89 cells ✓-ed to indicate compliance.*

How do we choose our compliance target? There's a rule of thumb that 90% will sustain fat loss or muscle gain. I looked far and wide for research supporting this and came up dry. In the end, it's a good starting point. Next consider the time sensitivity of your goals and how

---

*Each table has a maximum of thirty-five open cells. Each weekend day has two cells blacked out. That leaves thirty-three cells per week spread across three weeks (twenty-one days) or a total of ninety-nine opportunities to comply. 90% of ninety-nine is 89.1.

disciplined you can be. For an extreme example, if your goal is to lose five pounds in one week (it's possible), you have very little wiggle room and need to aim for near 100% compliance. If the time frame for your goal is further out, you have more leeway.

Also look closely at the constraints you identified when you were analyzing the Plan inputs. If you have dinner every Sunday at Mama's house, and it will destroy her if you don't eat her lasagna, but eating lasagna qualifies as noncompliance with your plan, you're starting off with 5% noncompliance right out of the gate.[*]

This brings us to my final suggestion on managing compliance. You'll be more successful reaching your goals if you plan ahead for noncompliance. It's better to know ahead of time which days and times you don't expect to hold yourself to the plan you created. You will also be more successful if you decide up front how your noncompliance will play out. For example, if you're going out for pizza and beer on Thursday, decide before you go what you'll order and how much you'll consume. Try to stick to this but don't beat yourself up if you fall off course. If you do, it seemed like a good idea at the time. Instead, try to learn something from the event and come up with strategies for the next time. Coaches are very good at helping with this stuff.

Compliance with Embedded Constraints

An embedded constraint contradicts the plan's guidelines but is inextricably tied to you. As you now know, foods with added sugar, refined carbohydrates, and alcohol are not covered by the mantras. But for many of us, these are some of the most pleasurable foods, so pleasurable that they are part of our lives. This plan wouldn't be *The Karma Sense Eating Plan* if it denied this. There are several strategies for addressing these cases.

---

[*] Three meals per day is twenty-one meals each week. One noncompliant meal represents 5%.

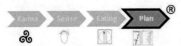

I'll be the guinea pig for this discussion. I like ice cream, and I like to have a drink now and then (as long as now and then is most nights around dinner time). I really would like to maintain my weight. With ice cream, I'd happily eat it every night but I can skip a few nights a week without having a tantrum. So I don't have it every night. On nights when I do eat it, I try to earn the ice cream by making sure my day is especially active. For alcohol, I usually have a drink or two most nights. My drink of choice is beer or red wine. I know that I don't tend to gain weight if I drink red wine. I now have habits for ice cream and alcohol that I can add to my Plan table. If I eat ice cream on a day when I did not meet my activity goal or if I have beer instead of wine, I understand these are noncompliance events.

And if I want to drop a few pounds? I adjust my plan to give up my embedded constraints until I reach my goal. I find this very manageable when I know it's for a finite period. Sometimes, it allows me to shake the habit altogether. French fries used to be one of my embedded constraints. I gave them up, as well as beer, to meet a goal and they both became bygone habits. Unfortunately for those good habits, my last startup's office was in Belgium where they make the best fries and beer in the world. I occasionally crave them now, but as noncompliance foods instead of embedded constraints.

You now have everything you need to build your own Karma Sense plan. If you're dying for additional detail, see the Appendix for some Karma Sense Eating planning tools. To close, let's look at one more example, but this time with a high specificity goal.

A High Specificity Example - Eat Veggie Chili, Billy

Billy is an aspiring scientist and computer enthusiast. As the Blue Power Ranger, he also controls the Triceratops Zord. Billy spends many late nights in his lab and sitting at the computer. Much like a triceratops, he is a vegetarian but lives on instant ramen and late night pizza delivery. Lately, Billy's less effective in battle. He leads a sedentary lifestyle except when he's called to action. With his lack of activity, his late hours, his stressful secret life, and his dependency on convenience foods, his belly is expanding.

Examining his vision and values, Billy decides he needs to be a more effective fighter of evil and nastiness. He wants to focus on gaining muscle and losing fat. His goal is to lose twenty pounds of fat while packing on five pounds of muscle within the next year. His only constraints are that he still wants to eat pizza every once in a while, he wants to eat mostly plants but is OK eating dairy and eggs, and his foods need to be convenient.

Billy's goal is high specificity. It will require nutrition planning that is beyond this book's scope. Billy's scientist brain enables him to develop a plan without the support of a coach, but he decides to depend on one because he can be absent minded and values a coach's motivational support. Also, while he may have the knowledge to manage his macronutrients, he really isn't that great in the kitchen. Together he and his coach develop a very specific plan that matches Billy's goal and body type. The plan tracks total calories, macronutrients, and syncs with *The Karma Sense Eating Plan*. Billy's Karma Sense Plan for each week looks like this:

Habit	Su	Mo	Tu	We	Th	Fr	Sa
Eat 1800 calories per day							
Eat 155 g of protein per day							
Eat 115 g of carbohydrates per day							
Eat 80 g of fat per day							
Only eat pizza on exercise days							
Walk to get pizza and groceries							
Resistance exercise 3 days/week.	■		■		■		■

Table 11 Billy's Karma Sense Compliance Tracker

As a vegetarian, Billy will have difficulty getting enough protein, so he works closely with his coach to devise meal plans. It involves eating more eggs and beans than he is used to, but it's worth it. Billy understands he needs to find alternatives to the refined carbohydrates he

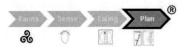

eats, but he can't give up the convenience they offer. His coach teaches him a cool technique to prepare a whole carb, high protein vegetarian chili on the weekend that will last several days in the refrigerator and can be dressed up to seem like a completely different meal every day. The chili also includes his vegetable servings for the week, which wasn't an explicit goal but a nice side benefit (you can find the recipe for "Mad Lib Chili" or "Billy Chili" in the Karma Sense Cooking section of the Appendix). Finally, Billy, who like most scientists believes in climate change, agrees to walk instead of drive to get the food he needs. This counts as his additional contribution to the greater good that he will reflect upon before meals. To help build muscle, Billy needs to perform resistance exercise three days per week. He blocks out the days he doesn't plan to exercise on his planning table.

Because Billy's plan is highly specific, it benefits from a more detailed set of actions. Also, since he has a specific time frame in mind, he will aim for 95% compliance. If he finds he is progressing faster than expected, he will throttle that down to 90% if it will help his mindset. It's possible that once he gets used to cleaner eating, he will not want to revert to the old habits that made him feel sluggish.

Billy is ready to roll. It's Morphin time!

What Gets You Excited?

I came up with the concept of *The Karma Sense Eating Plan* in a dream that jolted me awake. It was an exciting way to wake up. It put me on a path to some marathon writing over many nights so I could capture it all before I got distracted by something else.

Each time I released a new blog post, my excitement grew as I advanced that much further in explaining the entire process. The activity also allowed me to do many things that I love—write, talk about how food is remarkable, research nutrition and health, crack stupid jokes, etc.

This chapter, therefore, is somewhat anticlimactic for me as I hand the steps to leading a life of Karma Sense over to you. You can do this by:

- Getting a feeling for the building blocks—the components and mantras of the plan.
- Defining the destination you expect to reach by exploring your vision, values, and focus.
- Becoming in touch with your constraints—the non-negotiables, avoidables, and foibles.
- Settling on a goal.
- Identifying what and who you may need for support.
- Matching your goals to the most relevant and useful building blocks.
- Structuring your plan, including your compliance schedule.

But anticlimactic or no, I'm still excited. There's a lot of world-saving to do. The remaining pages of this book contain tools and reference material to help you on your way. But I don't want to end here. If you ever have any questions, comments, or just want to dig deeper into any details on this or related subjects, please contact me. I promise I'll be 100% engaged.

I went to sleep one night and something exciting happened when I woke up. I woke up with a superpower.

May you all wake up to something exciting!

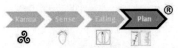

"When you wake up in the morning, Pooh," said Piglet at last, "what's the first thing you say to yourself?"

"What's for breakfast?" said Pooh. "What do *you* say, Piglet?"

"I say, I wonder what's going to happen exciting *today?*" said Piglet.

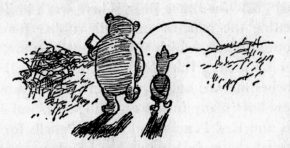

Pooh nodded thoughtfully.
"It's the same thing," he said.

Figure 51 Pooh — My First "Comic Book Superhero".[151]

Appendix

A Sample Mindful Eating Practice

Executive Summary

This section describes personal practices you can adopt to reacquaint yourself with the wonders and sensation of eating. It's offered as one of several techniques for mantra #1, Eat Slowly and Stop Before You're Full. The plan does not require that you adopt a mindful eating practice to take advantage of its benefits. The chapter describing mantra #1, Eat Slowly and Stop Before You're Full, offers other techniques. Also, a mindful eating practice can stand on its own. You can become a mindful eater without anyone accusing you of being part of that weird Karma Sense Eating gang that thinks they're so cool because they are healthy, happy and saving the world.

Mindful Eating Preparation

- Be sure you have no distractions (i.e., no TV, no reading, etc.). Dining companions are fine. This practice can be done individually, as a group, or individually within a group. If you're in a group and you're the only one practicing, let the others know. Many people can handle the progression of this practice while carrying on polite conversation at the same time. Others prefer not to. It's up to you. Do what works best.
- If you are doing this as a group, it's often more meaningful if it's done over a meal with which the group has some shared affinity. For example, a family who has a traditional meal or a group of friends at a favorite restaurant. Choose a leader to direct the activity.
- If at any time during this exercise, you find your mind wandering from the task at hand, acknowledge it, toss away the thought, and bring your focus back to the meal. Having your mind wander is normal and not an indication that you're doing anything wrong. When you notice it's happening, you're doing it right.

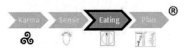

- Begin the practice when you're seated and your meal is placed in front of you. From that point forward, progress through the following sequence. Feel free to skip any steps that make you uncomfortable. Enjoy the experience.
- If you're having a multi-course meal, decide ahead whether you'll go through the process for each course or whether you'll single out a specific course.

Mindful Eating Progression

1. Make sure you're in a comfortable position.
2. Take a deep breath in and out and just accept whatever happens in the moment. Don't worry about your other senses at this time. If you smell something, don't try to process what it is. Just let it be.
3. Notice how you feel right now. Are you hungry? Is your stomach grumbling? How does the inside of your mouth feel? What is your general mood? Remember these feelings as you continue through the mindful eating process. You'll be asked to check in on these feelings again.
4. Move your nose as close as comfortably possible to your meal, close your eyes if you like, and take another breath to appreciate the aroma of the food you're about to eat. Do any smells stand out? Can you anticipate how the meal will taste? Are there spices and other ingredients that you easily recognize? Is the environment in your mouth changing? Is it getting drier? Are you salivating? If this is something you've eaten before, is there any difference in the aroma from your previous experience? When you're ready, move to the next step.
5. Examine your meal with your eyes and try to filter out your other senses. Notice the colors. Are you able to distinguish individual ingredients? Name them to yourself if it helps. If this is something you've eaten before, is there any difference in appearance from your previous experience?

6. Some food makes noise. Is your meal sizzling? Does it snap, crackle or pop?

7. Is this a food that you can politely touch or hold such as something you can eat with your hand? How does it feel? Is it hot or cold? Is it smooth or does it have texture? Does it leave any moisture or residue on your fingers?

8. Take another deep breath to take in the meal's aroma once again. Even though no food has entered your mouth, you are tasting what you are about to eat. While a great deal of flavor perception comes from the sense of taste, the sense of smell contributes the most. This is why food tastes differently when your respiratory tract is congested.

9. We'll now transition to tasting the food, but not at the expense of your other senses. Prepare to take your first bite, and make it slightly smaller than what you usual take. You're going to experience it for a longer time and that may be challenging if you take too large a bite.

10. Place the food in your mouth and move it around with your tongue before starting to chew. See if you can move it to make contact with your inner cheeks as well as the top, sides, and the underside of your tongue. Can you taste the individual flavors that your taste buds support? Can you distinguish the salty from the sweet? The bitter from the sour? Can you taste umami, the fifth flavor known as meaty or savory?

11. How does the food feel in your mouth?

12. Does the food smell any differently? Can you distinguish between the flavor that comes from your sense of taste and the flavor that comes from your sense of smell?

13. During this time, your saliva releases enzymes that begin to breakdown complex carbohydrates into simpler sugars. This will change the taste of your food while it's in your mouth. Can you sense the change over time?

14. Begin chewing and chew the food for as long as possible before swallowing. Notice the changes in flavor and the changes in

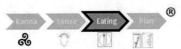

texture. Notice which teeth you use to chew depending on the consistency of the food. Keep chewing. Before you take your first swallow, your stomach begins to mobilize for digestion. Enzymes, bile, and other digestion assistants are secreted where necessary.

15. When you finally need to swallow, go ahead. Pause before you take another bite. It takes less than ten seconds for the bolus (the scientific name for a mass of food after it's swallowed) to reach the stomach. Wait about thirty seconds. In step three you were asked to note how you feel. Whether you were hungry. If your stomach was grumbling. How the inside of your mouth felt. What your general mood was. How have these feelings changed?

16. Repeat steps one through fifteen two more times. Each time, note if there are any differences in the feel, smell, and taste of what you're eating.

17. After three complete cycles, continue eating with smaller bites than usual but without concentrating on the distinct steps. Try to pay attention to all of your senses at once. Most important, try to eat more slowly than you usually do, and stay tuned to your hunger cues and your mood. Note if the food tastes any different from when you started. Pause your eating when you're no longer hungry. Wait five minutes and, as time progresses, notice if your hunger changes or if your mood changes.

18. If, at the end of five minutes you're still hungry, try eating a little more (three bites or so) and pause again. Continue this cycle until you're no longer hungry. Stop before you're full; you simply want to be satisfied.

19. Note how you feel fifteen minutes after you finished eating. Do the same one, two, and three hours afterwards.

This mindful eating progression is not something you need to do every time you eat for the rest of time. It's good to do with several different meals, varying the time of day, setting, alone or with others, home-cooked, at a restaurant, or carry out. When you finish, you may want to write notes about what's on your mind. Consider following this progression regularly, taking and comparing notes and examining any differences. Finally, you don't need to progress through the entire sequence with military precision. Just try the steps that appeal to you. If you want some crazy fun, live on the edge and do some of the weird stuff too.

Food Lists

Optimal Protein Sources

Protein	Note
Lean Meat	Beef, Chicken, Turkey, Pork, Bison, Venison. Grass and pasture fed preferred (see mantra #5)
Fish/Seafood	Wild caught from low in the food chain preferred Cold water fish helps with mantra #5
Eggs	Laid from cage-free chickens with natural diet preferred
Dairy	Greek yogurt, Cheese. High fat content can be an issue if weight loss is a goal
Plant Sources	Beans, Lentils, Peas, Nuts, Seeds, Quinoa, Soy, Buckwheat, Quorn, Seitan
Crickets, Insects and other Creepy Crawlies	Sustainable and nutrient-dense, while being inexpensive and low in calories. **Gross out your friends.**

Table 12 List of Optimal Protein Sources

Cruciferous Vegetables

Bok Choy	Chinese Broccoli	Mustard Greens
Broccoli	Cabbage	Napa Cabbage
Broccoflower	Kale	Radish
Broccoli Romanesco	Komatsuna	Rapini (Broccoli Rabe)
Brussels Sprouts	Kohlrabi	Rutabaga
Cauliflower	Maca	Savoy Cabbage
Collard Greens	Mizuna	Turnip Greens

Table 13 List of Cruciferous Vegetables from Brassica Genus. Most Research is Based on Brassicas.[152]

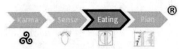

Starchy Vegetables

Beets	Parsnips	Taro
Carrots	Plantains	White Potatoes
Corn	Pumpkins	Winter Squash (Squashes other than Zucchini, Yellow and Petty Pan)
Green Peas (Note to Vegetarians: High in protein!)	Sweet Potatoes	Yams

Table 14 List of Starchy Vegetables.[153]

Best Omega-3 Fish

Albacore Tuna	Mussels	Sablefish/Black Cod
Anchovies	Oysters	Sardines
Arctic Char	Pacific Halibut	Wild Salmon from Alaska
Atlantic Mackerel	Rainbow Trout	

Table 15 Sustainable Fish, Seafood High in Omega-3s[154]

Types of Fats and Their Sources

| Type | Saturated | Polyunsaturated | | Monounsa-turated | Trans fat |
		Omega-3	Omega-6		
Source	Animal fats, tropical oils such as coconut	Fish, algae, some nuts and seeds	Vege-table oils, many nuts and seeds	Olive oil, avocado, many nuts and seeds	Innocent scientists who were kidnapped by shell corpora-tions created by aliens to destroy the human race
Good?	Yes	Yes	Yes	Yes	Never, no, blech!
Ratio to eat relative to other fats?	1/3	1/6	1/6	1/3	#DIV/0!
Typically Reduce or Increase?	Reduce	Increase	Reduce	Increase	Destroy!

Table 16 Types of Fats and Their Sources.

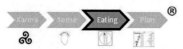

Dominant Fats in Nuts and Seeds

Nut/Seed	Saturated	Monoun-saturated	Omega-3	Omega-6
Almonds	4	32	0	12
Brazil Nuts	16	23	0	24
Cashews	9	27	8	8
Chia Seeds	3	2	18	6
Flax Seeds	4	8	23	6
Hemp Seeds	3	0	7	24
Hazelnuts	4	46	0	8
Macadamias	12	59	0	1
Pecans	6	41	1	21
Pine Nuts	9	23	1	25
Pistachios	5	23	0	13
Pumpkin Seeds	9	16	0	20
Sesame Seeds	7	19	0	31
Sunflower Seeds	4	19	0	23
Walnuts	6	9	9	38

Table 17 Dominant Fats in Nuts and Seeds (in grams per 100 grams of nuts)[155,156]

A Karma Sense Shopping List

A Karma Sense shopping cart is not limited to the foods on this list but it would contain plenty of the foods on this list.

Typical Grocery Aisle	Food	Type	Mantra	Comments
Produce	Avocado	Fat	#5	• Excellent source of monoun-saturated fats. • Can often be used instead of mayonnaise. • Avocado oil is a great alternative to olive oil on salads.
Produce	Banana	Fruit/Carb	#4	• Nutritional power house but high in calories. If the aim is to lose weight, avoid. • Consumption is driven by goal.
Produce	Berries	Fruit/Carb	#3, #4	• Excellent source of fiber. • Frozen berries are an excellent alternative to fresh. • Strawberries should be organic because they systemically absorb pesticides and fertilizers. Washing them doesn't remove these harmful agents. • Consumption is driven by goal.

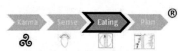

Typical Grocery Aisle	Food	Type	Mantra	Comments
Produce	Citrus Fruits	Fruit/Carb	#4	• Eat whole oranges or grapefruit. The fiber offsets the sugar content. Juice alone is mostly sugar.
Produce	Cruciferous Vegetables	Veg	#3	• See Table 13 for options.
Produce	Dark Leafy Greens	Veg	#3	• Collard greens, kale, and spinach are best if organic since washing does not remove pesticides and fertilizers. Organic versions are usually readily available in major super-markets • Other types such as arugula, beet greens, chard, dandelion greens and mustard greens are usually fine in their conventionally grown form.
Produce	Mushrooms	Veg	#3	• Excellent filler— Low in calories, high in micronutrients. No slouch where protein is concerned. • Great source of vitamin D and you can increase their vitamin D

Typical Grocery Aisle	Food	Type	Mantra	Comments
				content the same way you boost your own. Put them in direct sunlight the morning before using them. • To use as filler, process into very small pieces and add to most stir-fries, pasta dishes, or in meat-LESS meatballs (see in Appendix, Karma Sense Cooking) or meatloaves.
Produce or Canned Vegetables	Tomatoes	Veg	#3	• One of the few foods that are more nutritious when processed. • Canned tomatoes, tomato sauce and tomato paste all recommended. Watch for added sugar and salt. • Conventionally-grown cherry tomatoes are full of pesticides. Go organic for this variety only.
Dairy	Eggs	Protein	#2	• Aim for pasture raised or cage-free. This allows chickens to eat their natural diet and increases omega-3 content.

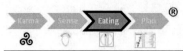

Typical Grocery Aisle	Food	Type	Mantra	Comments
Dairy	Greek Yogurt, Cottage Cheese	Protein	#2	• Best from organic cows or goats as these animals are not exposed to hormones, anti-biotics, and inflammatory diets. • Full fat or part fat versions are fine. They taste better than nonfat, are more satisfying, and good fat is your friend. • Avoid flavored varieties high in sugar. Make your own flavors by adding fresh fruit and nuts.
Meat	Fish	Protein/Fat	#2, #5	• See Table 15 for the best sources of omega-3s. • Frozen and canned are fine and sometimes superior choices for sustainability, nutrition content, and cost.
Meat	Lean Red Meat	Protein	#2	• Grass fed, wild, organic, and humanely raised is preferable. Animals raised this way are leaner and have higher omega-3 content. It's also

Typical Grocery Aisle	Food	Type	Mantra	Comments
				just good karma.
Meat	Poultry	Protein		• Cage–free, pasture-raised, and organic is preferred. Animals raised this way are leaner and have higher omega-3 content. It's also just good karma.
Packaged Foods	Beans, Peas, Lentils	Protein/Carb	#2, #4	• A Carb-olicious protein. • Dry beans taste better than canned, and you can control the salt content better. • Canned beans are more convenient than dry. • Mix it up. Try different types. • If vegetarian, consider beans as a protein. • Prepackaged hummus can have lots of added oils that add to calorie content. Also those oils are not always mono-unsaturated (the kind you need).

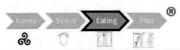

Typical Grocery Aisle	Food	Type	Mantra	Comments
Packaged Foods	Nuts/Seeds	Protein/Fat	#2, #5	<ul><li>A Fat-tastic protein.</li><li>Best when raw and unsalted but some don't enjoy them as much when not roasted.</li><li>Nut and seed butters are a fine source. Look for natural options vs. ones that contain partially hydrogenated oils (trans fats).</li><li>See Table 17 on the dominant fats in different nuts and seeds.</li></ul>
Packaged Foods	Oats	Carb	#4	<ul><li>If including grains in the diet, look for rolled or steel cut.</li></ul>
Packaged Foods	Olive Oil	Fat	#5	<ul><li>Use cold pressed extra virgin olive oil as it is the least processed.</li><li>Not meant for high heat cooking.</li><li>Store in refrigerator if not going to use within a few weeks of purchase.</li></ul>

Typical Grocery Aisle	Food	Type	Mantra	Comments
Packaged Foods	Quinoa	Carb	#4	• Although many consider quinoa to be a grain, it is actually a seed. • Unlike seeds, it is eaten in quantities similar to grains such as rice. It's also low in fat. • Quinoa is a better protein source than grains or most seeds because it provides a complete protein profile. But it is not a high protein source. To reach your daily protein goals you may need to supplement with other sources. • For best results, rinse quinoa before cooking otherwise it may have a soapy taste.
Packaged Foods	Spices	N/A	All	• Spices are high in micro- and phytonutrients yet low in calories. • See table of spice blends to give your creations a regional flair.

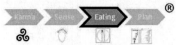

Typical Grocery Aisle	Food	Type	Mantra	Comments
Supplements	Fish or Algae Oil	Fat	#5	• If in pill form, store in the freezer to help you avoid fishy - burps.
Supplements	Greens Powder	Veg	#3	• If you aren't eating enough vegetables, these are a great way to reach your goal. They have a horrible taste. Best if blended in a smoothie with banana, nut butters and other ingredients with strong and pleasant flavors.
Supplements	Protein	Protein	#2	• Available from animal and plant sources. • Whey protein is the most popular animal source. • Pea protein is the most nutritious plant source. • Look for versions that contain limited or no artificial sweeteners and sugar alcohols.

Table 18 The Karma Sense Dream Team

Regional Flavor Blends

To give any dish (e.g., Mad Lib Chili or Meat-LESS balls that appear in Karma Sense Cooking section) a regional flair, add the following flavor combinations to taste. You normally would not add all of the spices listed and the proportions will vary.

Region	Herbs, Spices, Etc.
Cajun	Black pepper, cayenne pepper, garlic, oregano, paprika, thyme. Often available in a single package as Cajun Spice.
Chesapeake	Bay leaf, black pepper, cardamom, celery seed, cinnamon, cloves, ginger, mace, mustard, nutmeg, paprika. Together this is known as Old Bay. Common for seafood but good in other dishes too.
Chinese	Cashews, garlic, ginger, green onions or scallions, peanuts, rice vinegar, sesame oil, siracha, soy sauce or tamari, sesame seeds, sesame oil.
French	Basil, butter, garlic, herbs de Provence (which is a blend), marjoram, mustard, olive oil, rosemary, sage, tarragon, thyme.
Greek	Feta cheese, garlic, lemon juice or zest, onion, oregano, olive oil, rosemary, thyme.
Indian	Black pepper, cardamom, cayenne and other chili peppers, cloves, coconut milk, coriander, cumin, curry powder (blend), fennel, fenugreek, garam masala (blend), garlic, ginger, onion, turmeric, yogurt. Indian spice combinations are very subtle and hard to master so buying the blends is often a good bet.
Italian	Anchovies, balsamic vinegar, basil, crushed red pepper, fennel, garlic, lemon, marjoram, nutmeg, olives, olive oil, onion, oregano, parmesan cheese, parsley, red wine vinegar, rosemary, tarragon.
Jamaican	Allspice, brown sugar, cinnamon, cloves, crushed red pepper, cumin. Often available in a single package as Jerk Spice.
Japanese	Ginger, mirin, miso, rice vinegar, sake, soy sauce or tamari, rice vinegar, sesame oil, sesame seeds, wasabi.

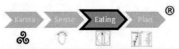

Region	Herbs, Spices, Etc.
Latin American	Chili powder, chili peppers, cilantro, cumin, garlic, onion, oregano.
North African	Anise, black pepper, cardamom, cayenne, cinnamon, cumin, ginger, harissa, lemon, mace, mint, nutmeg, sweet and hot paprika, saffron, sesame seeds, turmeric.
Thai	Cilantro, coconut milk, curry paste, fish sauce, garlic, ginger, lemon grass, onion, peanut butter, scallions, lemongrass, rice vinegar, soy sauce or tamari, Thai basil, and Thai chili peppers.

Table 19 Regional Flavor Blends

Karma Sense Cooking

Executive Summary

The following pages discuss reasons to cook more often, provide background on how I walk-the-talk, and offer practical strategies and cooking ideas that will work for almost anyone. In the end, don't over-think, use the Force and enjoy yourself.

Karma Science Cooking

Cooking your food is a Karma Sense way to achieve better health and happiness. I wouldn't say this without evidence. According to a recent study, people who cook at home most days of the week consume fewer calories, fewer carbohydrates, less sugar, and less fat than people who eat out often.[157] These results hold whether people who eat out opt for fast food or fine food; junk food or "health" food.[158]

Beyond the stuffy research, the intangible benefits of doing your own cooking are endless. It puts you in touch with the power of food. It gives you absolute confidence in the quality of the ingredients and preparation. It saves money and energy. It brings people together. It is one of the most practical creative outlets available in that you're going to eat anyway. And anyone can do it.

One benefit I don't claim, although it's also technically true, is that cooking burns more calories than outsourcing the cooking. It does indeed burn more calories than eating unlimited breadsticks at Olive Garden, about seventy-four to ninety calories per thirty minutes of cooking versus about thirty calories for just sitting (and further cancelled out by those unlimited breadsticks).[159] But one of the best parts about cooking is tasting your creation as you go along. In the end you probably aren't saving that many calories.

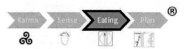

Wok the Talk

I've been cooking since I was a youngster. Both my parents worked, and I was a latchkey kid. Often if I wanted to eat, it was up to me. On weekends, I usually volunteered to cook lunch for my family. As I grew older, I wanted more control over which foods I put in my body. When I became responsible for paying for my own food, cooking was a cheaper option.

One year in college I spent a summer taking some extra classes to fill out my Psych requirements (I was going for a dual major in computer science and psychology). Durham, NC, was a ghost town during the summer. My food delivery job went on hiatus and I couldn't find another way to make money. I settled for the cheapest food I could find, which included a very large bag of dry lima beans. I ate a lot of limas that summer. They ended up in my boxed macaroni and cheese (the ramen noodles of the late twentieth century), mixed in with my can of tuna and, being ahead of my time, I even made meatless lima-burgers. I don't care what you're thinking right now; those lima-burgers tasted pretty darn good. In fact, I ate so many limas that when, for some unexplained reason, my housemates decided to assign each of us royal titles, mine was "Sir Rounded by Limas."* I'm guessing beer was involved but I'd been Missing In Action for awhile so I can't be sure.

After graduating and getting married, Mrs. H and I shared cooking duty. The Virginia girl and Jersey boy learned a lot from each other by working together. Once our kids were born, we took up the traditional path of stay-at-home mom and workaholic dad. I put my cooking skills on the shelf.

---

* Other housemates were "Sir Loin of Beef" (a blatant rip off of the *Bugs Bunny* cartoon "Rabbit Hood") and Duke of Marlboro.

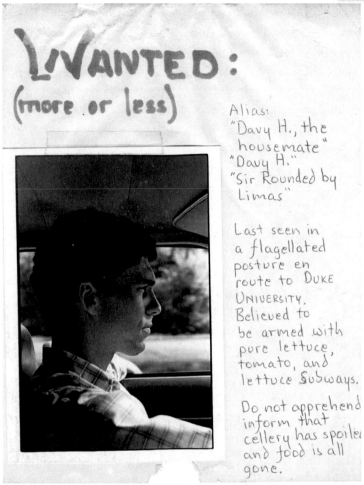

Figure 52 The Poster I Encountered on my Bedroom Door After Spending Some Time in Alternative Quarters at College[160]

Then a perfect storm occurred where I rekindled my interest in health topics, my wife went back to work, and I moved from a traditional office to a home office. This was a slippery slope for a workaholic since I now lived in my office. But knowing Mrs. H. would come home exhausted from her job, and that my two strapping boys had no patience, I had to put dinner on the table. Cooking became my mental commute—the transition time between work and home.

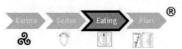

And to make things interesting, once my boys started college, their dietary preferences diverged. One became a vegetarian (and is now a dairy and gluten free vegetarian). The other is full-out gym-rat Paleo. Talk about inclusive? Try cooking a family meal for that crew!

But these challenges make cooking fun for me. I enjoy having a grab bag of ingredients thrown at me and having to create a meal. My favorite challenge is hearing about a client's craving for a beloved food that, due to a desire to be healthier, they avoid. I have fun collaborating with those clients to come up with alternatives and satisfy the craving. Whether it's peanut butter cups, ice cream, french fries, cheesecake, or brownies, making these foods just a little more nutritious is a blast. Or I'm easily entertained.

How to Approach Karma Sense Cooking

From my own informal poll, I learned that people avoid cooking because they don't have enough time or knowledge. Both challenges are easy to tackle. The ideas that follow are just that; they're ideas and not recipes. They're meant to jumpstart thinking about how to decrease the amount of cooking you outsource and take advantage of all the health and happiness benefits of doing it yourself. There are no pictures to make you feel bad that your creation isn't as beautiful as a photograph taken by a professional food photographer. I offer you lots of choice and options. This might intimidate some people. It shouldn't. Experiment and have fun. Don't give up if your first attempt isn't what you hoped. Instead, use your newfound mindful eating skills to learn what adjustments will help.

The cooking examples that follow demonstrate that, regardless of your obstacles to eating with healthful intention, there are strategies to work around them. The examples include:

- A lunch meal base that you can prepare ahead of time and suits just about any food tastes or constraints.

- A strategy for reducing meat consumption without eating more carbohydrates.
- Techniques for using low-carbohydrate vegetables as substitutes for grains and starchy vegetables.
- A way to balance your fat using a popular fruit in lieu of low-quality vegetable oils and saturated fats.
- The aforementioned and hopefully not overhyped roasted vegetable preparation.
- A homemade replacement for expensive protein and recovery bars. These are easy to make, and are suitable for the poor souls who can't eat nuts. Try and find a protein bar in your local store that doesn't contain nuts!
- A high protein and low-carbohydrate frozen dessert.

Mad Lib Chili (aka Billy Chili)

I call this Mad Lib Chili because "Make Your Own Adventure" Chili was too long and some people find the word "adventure" scary when it comes to putting things in their mouths. You can make Mad Lib Chili in large, multi-meal batches when you have time (such as on the weekend) and then quickly heat (if desired) when you're ready to eat. Mad Lib Chili doesn't always look pretty. But by definition, it tastes great because you're picking ingredients you enjoy.

The idea is to make a nutritious base with plenty of protein, vegetables and high-fiber carbohydrates that you can supplement with flavors when you're ready to eat. I've eaten mine with one or more of the following: siracha, salsa, soy sauce, fish sauce, flavored oils, muffaletta salad, tomato sauce, harissa, Cajun spices, guacamole, tzatziki, the colonel's secret blend of herbs and spices, and so on. If I'm in the mood for Italian, I add tomato sauce, basil, and oregano. If I want a Latin flair, I go salsa and guacamole. If I want Asian, I go siracha/soy sauce/fish sauce. North African—harissa. Greek—tzatziki. You get the idea. It's the shopping mall food court in a single bowl. In fact, if you start with a

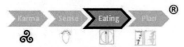

pound of protein, you should be able to create at least four meals for the cost of one at that same food court.

Ingredients

- Ground or small chunks of protein (ground beef, chicken, bison, tempeh, tofu, fish).
- Vegetables that you like.
- Beans or other legumes that you like or tolerate. If dry, prepare ahead of time.
- Other whole food carbs that are in line with mantra #4, Eat Whole Food Carbohydrates After Vigorous Exercise (rice, quinoa, sweet potatoes, beets). Prepare ahead of time.
- Fat to cook with (e.g., olive oil, butter, etc.).
- Herbs and spices of your choice.

Method

1. Chop your vegetables into bite size pieces or smaller.
2. If not using ground protein, chop or break the protein down to bite size pieces.
3. Put about a tablespoon of fat in a frying pan.
4. Put the firmer vegetables (carrots, broccoli, eggplant, onion, etc.) in first and stir them occasionally (or often if you want a little exercise).
5. As the firm vegetable soften, add the less firm vegetables (peppers, mushrooms, spinach, tomatoes, etc.).
6. Once the vegetables are at the desired texture, remove them from the pan and set aside.
7. Add a little more oil if your protein is ultra-lean. Once the pan reheats, throw in your protein.
8. Stir occasionally.

9. When protein is cooked through, add the cooked vegetables as well as beans, whole food carbs, and any herbs and spices you want until thoroughly mixed and warm.
10. You're done.

Notes

- This is a great lunch for the work week. Make it on the weekend and store it in a resealable container. Dish out your lunch size portion into a smaller container and you're set.
- I sometimes use canned tuna, salmon or even fresh fish as my protein. This might be a little hard core for some. When I make it with fish, I tend to make smaller portions so I don't stink up the refrigerator, or I add the fish within a few hours of the planned meal (e.g., in the morning when I pack a lunch).
- This chili is a great use for leftover vegetables from other meals. In fact, I often will incorporate leftover meat or other foods that will play well in this type of dish.
- The key to never getting tired of this meal is to vary your ingredients and sauces as much as possible. Be creative.
- Starchy vegetables like potatoes, sweet potatoes, beets, turnips, and winter squash can be terrific when incorporated into this meal. But they don't all pan-fry well. If you have a hankering for these ingredients, you can use the recipe for roast vegetables, described later in this section. Just be sure to roast them in advance and add them at the end with beans and other ingredients.
- Feel free to add cheese and eggs to this as well. Did I mention that you should be creative?
- The nutrition facts for this meal vary depending on the ingredients.

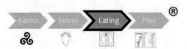

Meat-LESS Meatballs

Meatballs are a versatile way to get protein and other important nutrients. Most meatball recipes call for breadcrumbs or other carb-y filler to hold them together, to keep them moist, and to reduce the amount of actual meat needed. If you want to work around these carbs, you can do so thanks to the magic of mushrooms (not magic mushrooms though, unless you're into that sort of thing). Mushrooms can perform the same function as breadcrumbs. Furthermore, since mushrooms have a meatier taste and texture than breadcrumbs, you can use a lot of mushrooms without compromising flavor. This will save you money. Also, mushrooms are a great source of Vitamin D, and most of us don't get enough of that vitamin. Finally, it's a great way to eat less animal protein if that's your goal. Interested? Here's how to make Meat-LESS Meatballs; less carbs, less meat.

Ingredients

- 1 pound ground meat – fattier is usually better but don't worry if you prefer leaner meat like poultry
- 6 ounces mushrooms
- ½ onion, finely chopped
- 1 -2 cloves crushed garlic
- 1 egg
- Any herbs and spices you may like
- (Optional) 1 to 2 tablespoons of high quality oil (e.g., olive oil) or melted animal fats such as duck fat, lard or schmaltz (which I believe is Yiddish for chicken fat—no joke) only if using extra lean meat
- 1 tablespoon cooking oil

Method

1. Briefly chop the mushrooms in a food processor until they are somewhere in size between an individual bread crumb and a grain of rice.
2. Put first 6 ingredients (7 if using optional fat) in a bowl and mix by hand. While no one is watching, go ahead and build the mixture into funny shapes.
3. When thoroughly mixed, use a soup spoon to scoop up a hunk and place the mixture in your palm.
4. Put your hands together, as if you're going to clap, but not close enough to flatten the hunk of meat into a pancake. The distance between hands should be about an inch (2.5 centimeters).
5. Gently move your palms around until the hunk starts to become ball shaped.
6. Place the ball on a plate and repeat with another hunk until the giant mound of meat is converted to a dozen or so meatballs.
7. Heat the tablespoon of olive oil in a frying pan over medium heat.
8. Place the meatballs in the heated oil and let sit for 3 to 5 minutes.
9. If the bottoms start to turn a good "cooked meatball" color (brown), turn them over and continue until they're cooked all the way through and all sides are consistently browned.
10. Remove them from the pan when they are fully cooked and place on a paper towel to let the fat drain.
11. Refrigerate if not using immediately.

Notes

- If you don't have a food processor, you can chop the mushrooms with a knife, but you need to finely chop them. In my opinion, it's worth buying a cheap handheld food processor or immersion blender instead.

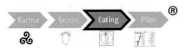

- You can add any of the spice combinations discussed in the Food List section of the Appendix to give the meatballs a local flair.
- Your meatballs can stand on their own or be used as the protein in Mad Lib Chili, on a sandwich, or with pasta. Even squash pasta.
- There are millions of recipes for true meatless (i.e. vegetarian) meatballs on the Interwebs. Meat-LESS meatballs are for people looking to reduce carbs or animal consumption.
- Add a couple of tablespoons of ground flax seed if you want to increase the fiber and good fat content.
- Using mushrooms instead of bread crumbs cuts calories by about 25% and carbohydrates by about 85% as compared to traditional meatballs.
- You can also use the mushroom filler trick with burgers and meatloaf.

Summer Squash Noodles

People usually approach pasta with one of two mindsets. Either they believe sauce enhances and elevates the pasta, or they believe the pasta is only a vehicle for the sauce. Regardless, traditional pasta is high in calories and carbohydrates and should be avoided if you're interested in losing weight or going gluten or grain-free.

People who belong to the "pasta is a sauce vehicle" camp have many options for pasta alternatives. They use noodles made from rice, quinoa, black beans, etc. They use spaghetti squash. Or they use the trendy new thing — zucchini or yellow squash. No substitute will ever satisfy those in the "sauce elevates pasta" camp. From my experience with victims of my cooking, a hybrid of zucchini or yellow squash noodles with standard wheat pasta is a good compromise.

To turn summer squash into pasta, you could buy a tool called a "spiralizer" that costs from ten to fifty dollars. A mandolin slicer is a more versatile tool that costs closer to fifty dollars and can also be used for slicing a variety of foods in many shapes and thicknesses. The mandolin's other advantage is the many hours of fun and entertainment you have learning to use it without slicing off your fingers. Or you can use a plain old vegetable peeler like you use to peel carrots. It costs about a buck and is useful for other tasks. What it can't do is cut your zucchini into all sorts of fun pasta shapes, but since none of these solutions duplicates the joys of Spaghetti-Os, who cares? I opt for the mandolin for its versatility and because the sight of blood doesn't scare me. If I'm lazy and not worried about the meal's appearance, I go vegetable peeler.

Regardless of the tool, many people prefer to use the fleshy part of the squash and toss the seedy portion in the middle. What you choose to do is your choice. The seedy portion contains more water and doesn't hold up well in some recipes.

There are many good websites that offer summer squash pasta (a.k.a., zoodles) recipes. Search the Internet for "zoodle recipes," "zucchini pasta recipes," or any other combination that makes sense. Also, if you just want to reduce your carbs without going low-carb, you can cut your normal amount of pasta by mixing in zoodles.

What follows is a very easy starter recipe that I inflicted on three pasta lovers with excellent success. It created a hearty and satisfying meal.

Ingredients

- 2 large zucchini or yellow squash
- A bunch of whole wheat spaghetti big enough to fit in the hole you make when the tip of your thumb touches the tip of your forefinger. Err on the small side.
- Any spaghetti sauce you like, preferably one that is low in sugar (e.g., less than five grams per serving)
- Meat-LESS Meatballs

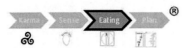

Method

1. Shred the squash into strips using the spiralizer, mandolin, or peeler.
2. Cook the spaghetti according to package directions. Shave one to two minutes off the suggested cooking time if you like your pasta *al dente*.
3. Simmer the sauce in a separate pot and throw the meatballs in to warm them up.
4. Drain the pasta when ready.
5. Stir the squash into the sauce just until it's mixed well.
6. Dish out the pasta.
7. Top the pasta with the meatballs and squash sauce.

Notes

- Summer Squash Noodles are a great way to increase your vegetable consumption a la mantra #3, Eat More Vegetables and Fruits.

Cauliflower Pseudo Carbs

Cauliflower can pinch hit for many carbs. You can simulate mashed potatoes. You can simulate rice. You can even simulate pizza crust, although I admit the pizza crust never comes close to fooling me. Here are methods for each. If you search the internet for "cauliflower" along with "mashed," "rice," or "pizza" you're bound to find something that may tickle your fancy. Assuming your fancy is ticklish.

Cauliflower Mash

Ingredients

- 1 head of cauliflower
- ¼ cup milk or milk substitute (e.g., almond, hemp, soy)

- 1 tablespoon of saturated fat (e.g., butter, coconut oil, ghee, lard)
- Whatever crazy herbs or spices you like in your mashed potatoes (garlic, chives, pepper, etc.)
- Salt and pepper to taste

Method

1. Cut florets off of cauliflower.
2. Cook cauliflower florets by either placing them in a steamer or metal colander and setting them over boiling water for twelve to fourteen minutes, or by putting them on a plate with a little water, covering the plate with wax paper, and microwaving at HIGH until the florets are soft (times vary, start with 3 minutes).
3. Drain cauliflower and place in food processor or the bowl of an immersion blender.
4. Add fat, milk, herbs, spices, salt, and pepper.
5. Blend until smooth.

Notes

- You can treat this like any other mashed potato recipe as far as flavors are concerned. If you like to make yours cheesy, go ahead.
- If you want to use fresh garlic, take a bulb and cut off the stem end. Drizzle the top with olive oil and wrap in foil. Bake at 400° F (200° C) for about 30 minutes. Let cool and squeeze the garlicky goodness into your "potatoes."
- If this recipe doesn't fool you and causes you to go off the wagon, then it may not be worth the effort. Find a way to build the real thing into your Karma Sense plan.

Cauliflower Rice

Ingredients

- One head of cauliflower

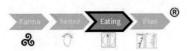

Method

1. Cut florets off of cauliflower. It's OK if you get more stem than with the mash recipe but don't include the stalk.
2. Break the florets into pieces with your hands.
3. Place everything but the stalk into a food processor and pulse at one second intervals until it's the consistency of rice. If certain pieces don't break down, don't panic. Proceed to next step.
4. Dump everything onto a plate and pick out any large pieces that didn't break down.
5. Place large pieces back in the food processor and give them another whirl. Repeat until bored.

Notes

- Cook this with 1 tablespoon of oil for about 5 minutes in a pan, and your rice is done. Eat as is or add to soups, stews, and salads that call for rice.
- Alternatively, you can make a stir-fried rice version. Just add the uncooked rice during the last 3 to 5 minutes of cooking other stir-fry ingredients.
- Some smart supermarkets are now selling cauliflower "pre-riced" at an incredible markup. Do what you want with this information.
- The rice may not be as convincing as the mash. If you're a non-believer, you can always go hybrid and mix in real rice. This combination would cut the carb count of your usual rice serving (mantra #4) and ramp up your veggie servings (mantra #3).
- If adding real rice still doesn't fool you and causes you to go off the wagon, it may not be worth the effort. Find a way to build the real thing into your Karma Sense plan.

Cauliflower Pizza

This recipe is not well suited to the novice cook. It requires advanced skills and, let's face it, it will never really be pizza. But don't let that scare you. It'll look good and it will taste good. It just won't taste like pizza. On my first try making this, the results looked horrible and tasted worse. I adjusted the method and ingredients and, on my second try, it looked like a bona fide homemade pizza. In no way did it taste like one but it still tasted pretty good. On my next try, I hit the target. It wasn't the pizza I grew up with in New Jersey, but it was tasty and nutritious nonetheless.

Before starting, be sure to have *cooking* parchment paper on hand. Accept no substitutes unless your fire insurance is fully paid. Also, the internet has many cauliflower pizza recipes. I advise against any that suggest a slow cooker and those that tell you to boil the cauliflower first. They just make the job harder without improved results.

Ingredients

- Cauliflower rice from above recipe, starting with about 2 pounds of cauliflower
- 1/3 cup soft, creamy cheese like cream cheese or soft goat cheese
- 1 egg
- Italian or other seasonings to taste
- Salt and pepper to taste
- Toppings: sauce, cheese, veggies, protein, etc.

Method

1. Preheat oven to 400° F (200° C).
2. Put the cauliflower rice in a bowl along with the remaining ingredients (except for toppings). For best results, mix with your hands and really work it to a doughy consistency.
3. Line a cooking pan with a layer of parchment paper. It can be round or rectangular.

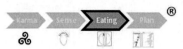

4. Spread the dough in the pan and flatten it out, so it's level. Aim for ¼-inch (7 mm) thickness. You can squeeze the edges a little higher if you want, so the sauce and cheese don't spill over the edge.

5. Place in oven for 30 to 40 minutes. You want the crust to become golden brown without over-cooking because you still need to add toppings and let it cook some more.

6. Add toppings and return to oven.

7. Check every 5 minutes or so to make sure toppings are heating the way you want and the crust is not burning.

8. Remove from oven, slice, and serve.

Notes

- The crust is really a veggie infused version of <u>Oopsie bread</u> but much more foolproof.[161]

- While low in carbs, don't fool yourself into thinking this is low in calories. With cheese in the crust and the toppings you include, there are plenty of opportunities to turn this into a calorie bomb.

- This crust will never fool you. But if you're more a fan of the topping than the entire pizza experience, if may be close enough to suit you.

Mantra #5 Slaw

Avocado is a great monounsaturated stand-in for cold recipes that call for saturated fats (e.g., mayonnaise, creamy dressing). This cole slaw recipe is easily modified.

Ingredients

- 6 cups shredded cabbage or other slaw-worthy vegetable
- 1 ripe avocado with flesh scooped out
- 2 tablespoons onion, finely chopped
- 3 tablespoons lemon juice

- ¼ cup small seeds (e.g., flax, sesame) or chopped nuts
- 3 tablespoons cilantro (If you don't think it tastes like soapy toilet water)
- Salt to taste

Method

1. Mix all ingredients in a large bowl until avocado is blended well.

Notes

- You can buy pre-shredded cole slaw vegetables.
- Up your game by using broccoli slaw or by creatively mixing up vegetables. Broccoli slaw is made from the stems and stalks that most people discard, but are perfectly edible. You also can use shredded asparagus, beets, carrots, summer squash, etc.

Roasted Veggies

Roasting vegetables until nicely browned (caramelized) creates a symphony in your mouth. Try this with as many different vegetables as you can. People who hate vegetables often join the "green" side once they've eaten a well-roasted vegetable. And it's so easy to do.

Ingredients

- As much cruciferous or root vegetable needed to feed everyone.
- Extra virgin olive oil
- Kosher or coarse Salt

Method

1. Preheat oven to 375 to 400° F (190 to 200° C)
2. Peel the vegetables if necessary and cut into bite size pieces.

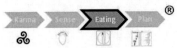

3. Place in bowl or roasting pan and splash with enough oil to evenly coat. Don't worry if you don't entirely coat veggies in oil. It's better to err on the light side.

4. Spread veggies evenly on roasting pan and sprinkle with kosher salt.

5. Check and stir every 5 to 10 minutes to see if they're roasted to your liking. You want the veggies to lightly brown or with a deep char if you roll that way.

6. When they look done, pull them out and serve.

Notes

- Total cook time should be 10 to 45 minutes. Bigger pieces and firmer vegetables take longer. For example, kale takes about 10 minutes. Brussels sprouts and broccoli take about 15 minutes. Potatoes take about 35 minutes.
- You may need to experiment to find your perfect vegetable and cooking time but it's worth it.
- If using kale, wash and dry the kale thoroughly and tear it into pieces about twice the size of a snack chip.

Mantra #4 Recovery Bites

You've completed some vigorous exercise and need something convenient and wholesome to eat. These make-at-home protein snacks are simple, versatile, delicious, and cheaper than protein bars or premixed shakes. Also, the base is nut free, so if you are sensitive or allergic to nuts, this can be your go-to recovery snack.

Ingredients

- 1 cup whole rolled oats
- 1 serving of your favorite protein powder; flavor and source (e.g., whey, protein, soy) is up to you
- 1 banana

Method

1. Add oats and protein powder to a food processor and coarsely grind, about 10 seconds.
2. Add banana, and run processor until the mixture is the consistency of dough.
3. Roll into balls between the palms of your hands. Makes about 12 ping-pong size balls.
4. Store in refrigerator in air tight container.

Notes

- Without any of the extras below and depending on the protein powder you choose, each ball is about 50 calories, 3 grams of protein, and 1 gram of fiber.
- If you start to form the balls and you find that too much of the mixture is sticking to your hands, put the mixture in the refrigerator and let it chill for about an hour. Don't chill for too long or the mixture becomes too crumbly.
- If the mixture is too crumbly, gently squeeze a ball's-worth in one hand and that should help it stick together.
- For added flavor, protein, and good fat, include 1 to 2 tablespoon of nut butter along with the banana.
- For added good fat and flavor, dust balls with unsweetened coconut flakes, or mix in coconut when you add the banana.
- As a special treat, stir high-quality dark chocolate chips into the dough between steps 2 and 3.

High Protein Ice "Cream"

This will never fly as a direct substitute for ice cream, but if you're craving a frozen treat, it can easily hit the spot.

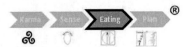

Ingredients

- 1 to 2 scoops of protein powder
- 1 to 2 tablespoons nut butter
- 2 to 3 ounces of milk or milk substitute

Method

1. Place protein powder and nut butter in the container you plan to freeze (and eat) from. I use a coffee mug.
2. Slowly mix in milk or milk substitute until the mixture reaches the consistency of pudding.
3. You can eat it now as pudding or freeze it for 30 to 60 minutes until it's the desired consistency. Don't let it go too long or it will become too hard to eat.

Notes

- Feel free to top with nuts or fruit before eating.

Plan Tools

The Plan component's chapter described how to design a plan that fits your goals. This section provides a series of tools to build your plan in a structured way.

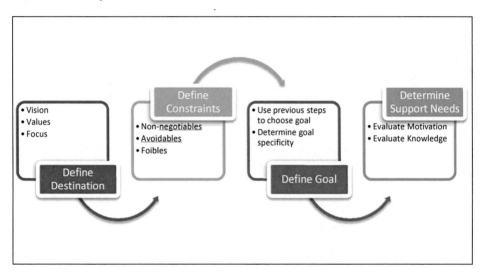

Figure 53 What You Should Know to Develop Your Karma Sense Plan

Step 1: Define Destination

This expanded set of questions defines each of the three dimensions (i.e., vision, values, and focus) of your end state.

Vision
• When you think about your best future, how far ahead do you look (e.g., five years, ten years, six months)?
• In that future, how will you feel mentally and physically?
• What will you be doing? Answer this one as completely as possible trying to address who, what, where, when, and how (e.g., who are you with?).
• How will you look and feel?
• What will achieving this vision make possible for you in your personal and professional life?
• What matters most to you in your health right now?

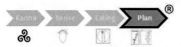

• How would making a change in this area make a difference in your life?
• What do you already know about how this area affects your life?
• If you don't change anything, what will your health and happiness be like in the future?

Table 20 Expanded Vision Questions

Values
• What really matters to you in life?
• What about your vision (from Table 20 Expanded Vision Questions) stands out as a reflection of what matters to you?
• What strengths do you have that will help you achieve the vision?
• What improvements do you need to make to achieve the vision?

Table 21 Values Questions

In addition, you can perform the following exercise. Review each of the values listed below. Select the five or so that are most important to you and rank them from most to least important. Don't worry if some of them seem to overlap or if you don't understand what one means. Take your best guess. What you end up with should reflect the answers to the questions above.

Acceptance	Dependability	Inner Peace	Mindfulness
Accuracy	Diligence	Integrity	Moderation
Achievement	Duty	Intelligence	Monogamy
Adventure	Ecology	Intimacy	Music
Art	Excitement	Justice	Nonconformity
Attractiveness	Faithfulness	Knowledge	Novelty
Authenticity	Fame	Leadership	Nurturance
Authority	Family	Leisure	Openness
Autonomy	Fitness	Loved	Safety
Beauty	Flexibility	Loving	Self-Acceptance
Belonging	Forgiveness	Mastery	Self-Control
Caring	Freedom	Order	Self-Esteem
Challenge	Friendship	Passion	Self-Knowledge

Comfort	Fun	Patriotism	Service
Commitment	Generosity	Popularity	Sexuality
Compassion	God's Will	Power	Simplicity
Competence	Gratitude	Practicality	Solitude
Complexity	Growth	Protect	Spirituality
Compromise	Health	Provide	Stability
Confidence	Honesty	Purpose	Tolerance
Contribution	Hope	Rationality	Tradition
Cooperation	Humility	Realism	Vitality
Courage	Humor	Responsibility	Virtue
Courtesy	Imagination	Risk	Wealth
Creativity	Independence	Romance	World Peace
Curiosity	Industry		

Table 22 List of Values[162]

When examining your values, take the time to reexamine the Save the World Model.

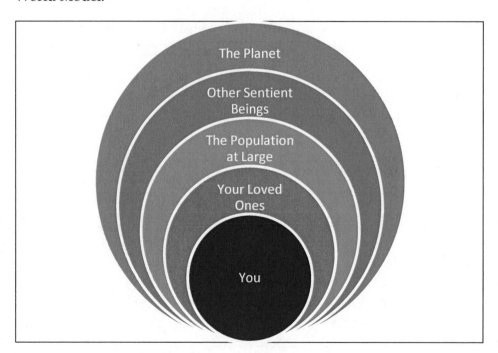

Figure 54 The Save the World Model

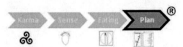

If you overlay the values you've identified onto each one of the possibly affected constituencies in the Save the World model, you can hone in on which good deeds may move you closer to saving the world. For example, if you value your leisure, then the "You" circle is an important aspect of your world-saving view. If you value justice, then the Population at Large is a good target.

Focus
If you were going to make a change, what would it be?
When thinking about the improvements you want to make,
• Which are most important in the short term?
• Which are most important in the long term?
• Which are the most difficult to achieve?
• Which are achievable within the time frame of your vision?
• How motivated and willing are you to make the necessary changes?
• Which changes are you most confident about making now?
• How would you describe the changes so they become discrete actions that drive better health and happiness?

Table 23 Expanded Focus Questions

Step 2: Define Constraints

Here is what to ask to surface your constraints.

Non-negotiables
• What foods will you never eat because they violate some value or because the thought of them ties your stomach in a knot?
• What foods must be included in your diet because the thought of never eating them makes you sad, lonely, scared, or violent?
• What aspects of your life complicate your eating habits, such as travel, shift work, traditional family meals, or living next door to Five Guys?
Avoidables
• What foods present a value conflict (e.g., you like a food, but it violates one of your principles)?

• What foods would you like to eat more often but don't due to some limitation in your environment (e.g., you want to eat more broccoli but you haven't found a preparation that you like)?
• What foods do you think you should eat less often or believe you can reduce your consumption of, but just haven't done so yet?
• What situations do you typically face that challenge your discipline or self-control (e.g., you can't walk past a coffee shop without buying a giant coffee milkshake and there is a coffee shop on every corner)?
Foibles
• What unique or uncommon beliefs or habits do you have that impact how and what you eat?

Table 24 Constraint Questions

Constraints Journal

Significant self-reflection provides a great way to surface your constraints. This can be difficult for some people. You can use journaling to assist in this process. Many people know the concept of food logging. When attempting to track calories and macronutrients, journaling can be a real drag. But it can be truly eye-opening if you do it with an eye towards what you won't eat or, conversely, what you don't refuse. It's not as annoying as food logging, although strangers may decide to keep their distance as they watch you take notes while you're eating. Here is a step-by-step process to pursue this method. It's not the only way but if you don't know where to begin, this proposal will help.

Setup

It's important to keep your constraints journal handy at all times. Identify your journal medium (e.g., notepad, smartphone, etc.) and make an agreement with yourself to use it every time you make a food-related decision. The perfect time period for this kind of exercise is three to seven days. If you don't journal each day of the week, try to cover all the

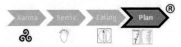

kinds of days you typically experience (e.g., work and weekend, classes and no classes, house arrest and probation, etc.).

Method

You face many food-related choices during the day. These include what to eat, what not to eat, what to buy for later, what to throw out, etc. Your mission is to record each of these decisions in your journal for later analysis. Capture the following decisions throughout the chosen period. Note the date and time for each decision.

- Each time you decide to have a meal, what drives that decision?
    - Hunger?
    - The clock?
    - Someone offering food?
    - Anything else?
- How do you decide what to eat?
    - When reviewing a menu, what drives your choice of one item over the other?
    - When preparing a meal for yourself, with or without others, what determines your choice for what to eat?
    - Did you consider other options that you ultimately did not select? Why did you choose something else?
    - When someone offers a specific meal with no options, how do you deal with the situation? Include the following considerations:
        - "This is something I enjoy and will eat."
        - "This is something I usually enjoy but am not in the mood for but will eat out of courtesy."
        - "This is something I enjoy but am not in the mood for so will only eat some or none."
        - "This is something I do not like but will eat out of courtesy."

- "This is something I do not like so will only eat some or none."
- "I have never had this before but will give it a try."
- "I have never had this before and, um, no."

- As you begin and continue eating what drives each of these decisions?
  - How you'll eat it (e.g., hands, utensils, etc.)?
  - What you'll eat on (e.g., plate, bowl, wrapper)?
  - Is there any reason you chose the particular eating equipment you are using?
  - How did you choose the arrangement of your meal?
  - What position will you be in (e.g., at a dining table, standing, at your desk)?
  - How quickly will you eat?
  - When will you decide you are finished eating?
- What do you do with any leftovers and why?
- What drives your decision not to eat even if you're hungry?
- What drives your decision not to eat even if it's meal time?
- When shopping for food, how do you decide what to buy?
- What inspires you to try a new food?
- How do you decide to dispose of food that you've stored or saved?

Analysis

To analyze your journal, review your notes in light of the constraint questions in Table 24 Constraint Questions. This will provide better insight to your constraints.

Realize, in the end, these constraints may have no effect on your Karma Sense Eating Plan implementation. But you don't want to develop a plan only to discover it was doomed to fail from the start because you didn't include these constraints in your thought process.

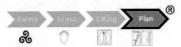

You now have, as a result of the destination and constraint exercises, a complete inventory of everything that matters in your life. It should include your thoughts on:

- How active and rested you want to be.
- How you want to nourish your body and your soul.
- Who matters to you.
- Where you want to be physically and mentally.
- How you want to spend your time.
- Any themes that tie all these together

Step 3: Define Goal

Before you even started reading The *Karma Sense Eating Plan*, you possibly knew what improvements you wanted to make in your life for greater health and happiness. Often, after completing the destination and constraint exercises, new priorities begin to surface. This is one of the great aspects of going through those exercises. Whether you're sticking to your original goal, refining it, or going with something new, once you decide on the goal, assess its specificity to decide whether you can accomplish it alone or if you need support. Table 25 How to Analyze Your Goals, shows you the benefits and risks of different goals depending on how specific they are.

Goal Specificity	Examples	Flexibility	Ease of Tracking	When You Can Go It Alone	When to Seek a Coach
Low	I want to be healthier, happier, and save the world.	High	Low	You're satisfied with your health and the plan feels like a positive step	You know you want to make specific improvements but you can't define them

Goal Specificity	Examples	Flexibility	Ease of Tracking	When You Can Go It Alone	When to Seek a Coach
Medium	• Lose weight. • Maintain weight and be healthier. • Gain weight in the form of muscle. • Manage stress. • Improve attitude. • Feel like I'm making a meaningful contribution.	Medium	Medium	You are highly disciplined and motivated; you will not get discouraged by short-term setbacks	You need help with motivation or discipline; any setback may cause you to revert to undesirable habits
High	• Improve body composition to 15% body fat. • Be active with grandchildren in your sixties and seventies. • Climb Mt. Everest within five years.	Low	High	You are highly motivated, disciplined and knowledgeable about what you need to do to reach your goal.	You lack the knowledge to achieve your goal regardless of how motivated or disciplined you are.

Table 25 How to Analyze Your Goals

To test whether a high specificity goal is truly realistic, consider using the well-worn SMART system. Tons of resources are on the internet, but to summarize it here, SMART stands for:

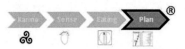

- Specific – you should be able to answer the who, what, where and why questions.
- Measurable – you should be able to identify the metrics you will use to demonstrate and evaluate your progress towards your goal.
- Achievable – your goal should be challenging yet realistic.
- Relevant – your goal should be something you care about.
- Time-Bound – your goal should have a timeframe in which it is achieved.

Step 4: Determine Support Needs

Now that you understand the risks and benefits of your goal, it's time to decide whether you'll need or want help. Here's the table presented in the Plan component description. It is only relevant if you want support.

How High Is Your		Motivation	
		Low	High
Knowledge	Low	Health Coach	Nutrition Coach
	High	Health Coach	Wild Card

Table 26 What Kind of Support Should You Get?

Step 5: Determine Which Components and Mantras Apply

The following table summarizes the considerations for which components and mantras apply to your goals as presented in the Plan component.

Building Block	Summary	Recommendation	Comment
Karma	Do a good deed.	Implement this component early.	Build an intentional good deed into your routine before worrying about how it can drive better eating habits.

Building Block	Summary	Recommendation	Comment
Sense	Link your good deeds and other "happiness catalysts" to your eating routine.	Defer implementing this unless you're a "big banger" or you're opting not to adopt the Karma component.	If you're adopting the Karma component, allow that habit to become ingrained before adding this one. Don't try too much behavior modification at once. However, if you want to focus on mantra #1, consider adopting this component along with Karma and mantra #1 and stopping there for now.
Eating			
Mantra #1	Eat Slowly and Stop Before You're Full.	Adopt as soon as possible.	Has no downside unless it interferes with a goal to gain weight (build muscle). May be hard to implement without including the pre-meal ritual of the Sense component.
Mantra #2	Eat Protein in Every Meal.	Implement along with mantra #3 and #5.	Great mantra to support losing weight or building muscle. For optimal health, it's helpful to consume the micro- and phyto-nutrients in plant food and be sure to get the balance of fats from non-protein sources.
Mantra #3	Eat More Vegetables and Fruits.	Best mantra to adopt in isolation or with others.	High value nutrition at minimal caloric cost.

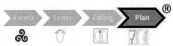

Building Block	Summary	Recommendation	Comment
Mantra #4	Eat Whole Food Carbohydrates After Vigorous Exercise.	This mantra can be adopted in isolation.	The key to this mantra is timing carbohydrate consumption soon after exercise so that your body processes optimally. Unless you're an elite or endurance athlete, carbs aren't necessary after vigorous exercise. If you choose to exercise and not follow with carbs, you're still honoring this mantra.
Mantra #5	Eat Good Fats Daily and Balance a Variety of Good Fats.	This mantra is best adopted in conjunction with mantra #2.	If adopting this mantra in isolation, be sure to understand your current fat intake and adjust accordingly. If adopting this mantra in conjunction with others, be sure that your fat balance matches your new habits.

Building Block	Summary	Recommendation	Comment
Plan	Define a roadmap for how you will honor *The Karma Sense Eating Plan*	Navigate through the process in this appendix and map your plan with the tools provided.	There's nothing wrong with taking on *The Karma Sense Eating Plan* without adopting this component. The Plan component is there so you see progress and stay motivated. But honestly, if you're not interested in adopting the Plan component, why the heck are you even reading this section?

Table 27 Determine What Mantras and Components Apply

Step 6: Map Your Plan

Here is a blank table you can use to build out a plan. This is similar to what Kimberly and Billy used in each of the examples in the Plan description.

Week _____

Habit	Su	Mo	Tu	We	Th	Fr	Sa

Table 28 Blank Planning Template

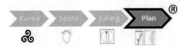

Step 7: Factor in Compliance

There are three main considerations to factor in compliance.

Factor 1: Identify Your Target Compliance

Unless you already understand what your target should be, I recommend that you start with 90%. The percentage should be higher if your goal is particularly aggressive (but still realistic!). The percentage can be less than 90% if your timeframe can tolerate slower progress. Your initial choice is not cast in stone; you can adapt it as needed.

Factor 2: Acknowledge Your Embedded Constraints

You should have identified your constraints in the constraint exercise in Step 2. Now is the time to work them into your plan. Without acknowledging your constraints, your plan is not realistic. If you feel you don't need to include them, they're not really embedded.

Factor 3: Plan for Your Remaining Times of Non-compliance

At this point, you understand what you will do to comply and your target compliance percentage. You've also mapped those times when compliance is not possible due to embedded constraints. If any non-compliance opportunities remain, plan for them. It's always best to plan the "when" and "what" of non-compliance ahead of time because you'll be less likely to overindulge.

In the description of the Plan component, I include a hypothetical example of you having dinner every Sunday at Mama's house and have no choice but to eat her noncompliant lasagna. In that example, you were starting off at a maximum of 95% compliance right out of the gate. If your target compliance was 90%, you can have one additional noncompliant meal per week.

Of course, you have the other option to exercise two hours before heading to Mama's house or to convince Mama to make her lasagna with thinly sliced winter squash or eggplant in lieu of pasta. I give the latter a low probability of success.

Super Wowie Bonus Fun

The Super Wowie Bonus Fun section is chock-a-block filled with additional information to support your life of Karma Sense. Like Jell-O to a full stomach, it fills in the cracks with topics that are relevant to the overall plan, but had no right being discussed in the body of the book.

Alcohol and Its Role in Karma Sense Eating

OK. I kicked this beer can down the road long enough. Time to face *The Karma Sense Eating Plan*'s drinking problem. The challenge of including alcohol in the plan is that I don't really consider its consumption as "eating" (even when consumed as Jell-O shots.). Alcohol consumption is a recreational activity that, when used conventionally (and not through enemas, which apparently is a "thing," but I suggest you don't search Google Images for it), happens to use the same body parts as when you eat. The following paragraphs discuss the role of alcohol when living a life of Karma Sense.

Many people misconstrue alcohol as a type of carbohydrate. This is wrong. Alcoholic beverages usually contain carbohydrates, but the alcohol itself is not a macronutrient. Unlike protein, carbohydrates, and fats, you cannot survive on alcohol. Consuming alcohol in moderation however, has proven health benefits. Red wine is especially regarded as having positive health effects. Studies on other types of alcohol suggest a positive correlation but they are confounding.[163]

Moderate consumption means one drink or less per day for women and two drinks or less per day for men. Sorry ladies, I sincerely wish there was something I could do about that. A single serving is the equivalent of twelve ounces of beer (350 ml), five ounces of wine (150 ml), or one-and-a-half ounces (45 ml) of the hard stuff.

People looking to manage their weight through a low-carbohydrate diet should curb their alcohol consumption. Although alcohol is not a carbohydrate, it contains seven calories per gram vs. the four calories per

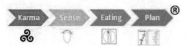

gram for carbohydrates. Also, the body tends to give alcohol priority over fats or carbs when burning energy. So even if you choose a low-carb alcoholic beverage, you are defeating the purpose if you're hoping to lose fat by managing carbohydrates.

The table below provides guidelines on the carbohydrate content of your beverage of choice (My name is Davey H and I am a table-a-holic).

Type	Carb Range Per Serving (in grams)
Beer	3-20
Wine	2-8
Liqueur	10-25
Hard Stuff	Trace

Table 29 Alcoholic Beverages and Typical Calorie Counts.

Note that, the sweeter wine and liqueur taste, the more carbs they contain. Also, if you're drinking the hard stuff with mixers, the sugar in the mixer counts. Yes, diet mixers don't usually have carbohydrates. They have artificial sweeteners that are gross. Finally, when cooking with alcohol, the alcohol itself burns off, reducing the calories. The amount burned off depends on how much you start with, cooking methods, and cooking duration.

Alcohol absolutely has a place when leading a life of Karma Sense. As noted earlier, I drink a glass or two of wine on most nights as well as the occasional beer. But please, drink Karma Sensibly.

Don't Waste Your Time Exercising

Executive Summary

In the movie *There's Something About Mary,* our hero (Ted) picks up a hitchhiker on his way to find the love of his life. During the drive, a conversation similar to the following takes place.

Hitchhiker: *You heard of this thing, the 8-Minute Abs?*
Ted: *Yeah, sure 8-Minute Abs. Yeah, the exercise video.*
Hitchhiker: *Yeah, this is going to blow that right out of the water. Listen to this...7...Minute...Abs.*
Ted: *Unless of course, someone comes up with 6-Minute Abs.*
Hitchhiker: *No! Not 6! I said 7! Who works out in 6 minutes?*[164]

It's a cheeky title, I know. Exercise is not a waste of time, yet people give lack of time as a common reason they don't exercise. Granted, the current official recommendations for exercise don't help. The American Academy of Sports Medicine and U.S. Department of Health and Human Services each have *minimum* recommendations for exercise that add up to about four hours per week.[165,166] These are minimums! Depending on your goals and current state, you may need more. With intimidating recommendations like this, of course people don't even try. For many, the thought of spending an hour at a time, four days a week on an elliptical at the gym is unpleasant and unlikely. It sounds so boring, I'm falling asleep simply writing about it.

This section offers solutions for optimizing exercise when you have limited time. The techniques I discuss won't necessarily get you to the optimal level of five to seven hours a week, or even the minimum of four, but it's a start. Research shows you don't have to complete the full four hours to reap benefits.[167] Furthermore, once you start seeing results from your exercise routines, you may find it easier to continue and even increase your exercise volume. While you may not achieve seven minute abs, you can make significant progress in as little as eight

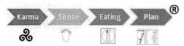

minutes. But before we get to this little secret, I'll once again drag you through a bit of science.

Definitions

- Steady State Exercise - is what you're doing if you exercise on a cardio machine (e.g., treadmill, recumbent bike, elliptical, stair climber) for thirty to sixty minutes at a nearly constant speed and resistance. Some people actually attempt this kind of exercise in an environment known as "outdoors" using equipment known as "the street." Theoretically this can also be done with calisthenics like jumping jacks, pushups, or even jump ropes but no one seems to do these kinds of things at thirty-minute clips.

- High Intensity Interval Training (HIIT) - An exercise routine that involves performing one or more exercises at full speed for brief periods alternated with brief periods of slower activity or full rest.

- Aerobic Exercise - Exercise that is not highly intense and depends <u>mostly</u> on the body's intake of oxygen to burn body fat as energy. Steady state exercise is primarily aerobic.

- Anaerobic Exercise - Higher intensity exercise that depends more on immediately available forms of energy in the body (ATP, sugar). These forms of energy are available to your body in limited quantities without requiring the oxygen you breathe. But remember, you need to breathe for other reasons too so don't try and hold your breath when doing anaerobics. If you get the gist of what I'm talking about and remain interested, this is the time to apologize to your high school biology teacher because that's something else you needed to know. HIIT depends heavily on anaerobic energy.

- Resistance Exercise - Activity that involves your muscles contracting against a force that opposes the motion (e.g., weight training) with the expectation of increases in strength, tone, mass, and endurance. These are anaerobic exercises that stimulate skeletal muscle fitness more than cardiac muscle fitness.

HIIT Me With Your Best Shot

There is a near religious debate among fitness fanatics about which exercise protocol reigns supreme.* If you hang with these people, you'll hear weight lifters disparaging the runners and runners disparaging weight lifters. These folks need to get lives. The discussion in this section doesn't make the case for HIIT as the superior choice. Instead, it explains how people who are intimidated by the time commitments required for exercise can benefit from HIIT. Ideally, your exercise routine would consist of steady state, HIIT, and resistance training. One of the key advantages of HIIT training is that you receive many of the benefits of all three.

Assuming you're clear on what steady state is (and if you're not, just read the definition above because that's all you need to know), let's dive a little deeper into HIIT.

HIIT first came to light in the 1990s after a study led by Izumi Tabata compared the fitness improvements between two groups of exercisers following different training regimens.[168] A steady state group worked out for one hour five times a week. The HIIT group exercised at maximum intensity for twenty seconds followed by ten seconds of rest. This group cycled through this sequence eight times for a *total of four minutes of exercise per day*. HIIT exercise was done four days a week with the addition of one steady state session. At the end of the study, the results showed similar gains in aerobic endurance capacity for each group. In addition, the HIIT group's anaerobic strength improved as well.

---

* For you *Iron Chef* fans.

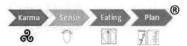

Imagine achieving the same results in 25% of the time! These results kicked off a nearly infinite number of follow-up studies on how HIIT regimens affect general fitness. And while these studies toned down the hype, the case for HIIT remains impressive. Perhaps most interesting, study after study shows that *when it comes to burning fat and building muscle, HIIT is superior to steady state exercise.*[169,170] I think I need to say it again. *You burn more fat and build more muscle by exercising in short repeated bursts than you do through long workouts at a sustained pace.* This doesn't mean that HIIT is the best style of exercising. The best style of exercising is the exercise you actually do. And there are cardiovascular benefits from steady state exercise that don't surface with HIIT.

Exercise With Karma Sense

So, how do we use this information practically? It depends. Your activity plan needs to reflect your wellness goals. Your best option is to adopt a variety of exercises. That said, here are some general guidelines.

If You're Not Currently Aerobically Fit

If you haven't exercised for a long time or if your heart rate per minute after a period of sustained rest is above the mid-seventies, focus on steady state training to improve your aerobic fitness. Since I don't want you to waste your time exercising, try some of the following ways to exercise productively:

- Take the stairs more often. This doesn't mean you should walk all four flights to get to your fourth-floor office on day one. Instead take the elevator up two stories and walk the rest. Work your way up to the full four flights.
- Walk up an escalator or along a moving walkway.
- Park your car twice the distance from the entrance to your destination as opposed to searching for the closest spot.

According to this <u>study</u>, you'll likely get to your destination faster too.[171]

- When you have to have an important discussion with others, talk to them while walking.
- Adopt some of the <u>Healthy Transportation</u> practices I posted on my website.[172]

With all of these practices you're doing something you would do anyway. The net effect on your time is minimal and comes with a huge payback. Once you've built up your aerobic fitness, you can increase your intensity

Add HIIT to Your Workout Routine

There are many ways to perform HIIT. The Tabata protocol is a start. Over time you should lengthen your high intensity periods as well as the duration of the overall routine. The best part about HIIT is that you can do it with or without equipment. You can also integrate strength and resistance training. Here are some ways I integrate HIIT into my fitness regimen.

- **Tabata** – I usually cycle or walk to get to my gym. On those occasions when I drive, I don't get the steady state workout I usually do. To compensate, I do two Tabata rounds on the rowing machine. No cardio machine in the gym matches the rowing machine for an overall workout. Also, no cardio machine is more boring. But I can tolerate just about anything for eight minutes, even *The Big Bang Theory*. And eight minutes of Tabata on a rowing machine is a hard workout.
- **Travel** - When I travel for work, I don't sleep as much, I don't interact with my family as much, and I don't have as many distractions. So I usually sneak in some extra workouts. On days when I don't do weights, the extra workout usually consists of thirty minutes on a bike or elliptical. I put my music on shuffle

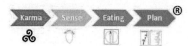

and with each song change, I alternate between high intensity and rest. This routine can lead to some long high intensity rounds. That's why *In A Godda Da Vita* no longer appears on my playlist. More realistically, you could push hard for ninety seconds and slow for sixty seconds, or use some other combination that works with your fitness level. I often read while I do this. Since most hotels have TVs in their exercise area, I could just as easily watch TV. As an aside, most people's anaerobic energy supply runs out after about ninety seconds, so high intensity work that lasts more than two minutes is rarely as intense as you think.

- **HIIT As Your Only Exercise** – During the winter of 2015, to "eat my own dog" food (mantra #2, Eat Protein in Every Meal), I decided to forgo my usual weight and gym routine for an at-home body-weight-only HIIT routine. This happened over the holidays and, like everyone else, I gained weight. In December, I did a different HIIT routine three days a week. You can easily find these routines on YouTube. Each lasted about thirty minutes. Since every routine differed, I had a full body workout and never got bored. In January, I found one routine that I stuck to. It had some crazy exercises that were challenging to master but had great results. One exercise combined a one-armed push up with a simultaneous horizontal jumping jack. It took me most of the month to master it. Another exercise that I never mastered on my best day, made me look like the least coordinated Rockette at Radio City Music Hall. Regardless, by the end of those two months I lost all my holiday weight with a total investment of ninety minutes of exercise per week. And I did these exercises in my home or hotel room with no equipment.

So, what are your reasons for not exercising? Do you not have time? Do you find exercise boring? Do you lack motivation to go to the gym? How about "I never see results"? HIIT may be the solution. And if it isn't, I bet we can find one.

Exercise has well documented benefits beyond the scope of this book. Combining HIIT into your routine provides a great way to honor mantra #4, Eat Whole Food Carbohydrates After Vigorous Exercise.

Full Disclosure: I am not a doctor and suggest you consult one if you are not currently exercising and you're considering HIIT.

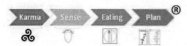

You Are Not "N" - The Role of Research in *Your* Karma Sense Eating Plan

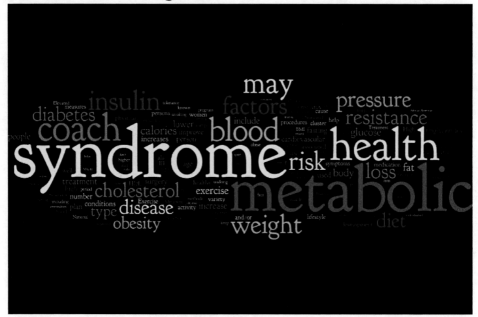

Figure 55 The Magic 8 Ball Says: The Future of Your Health is Hazy. Try Again Later

Executive Summary

As much as I depend on research to support the claims I make in *The Karma Sense Eating Plan*, I'm well aware that health and medical studies often add to the confusion. For example, if you try to follow all of the advice that comes from research, what would your day look like? Is it even possible to do? Should you worry about dietary cholesterol or can you eat all the eggs you want? This section provides background on the challenge of applying general medical research to your personal health.

There are Many Different Ways to Perform Research

Some research methods use subjective measures and others use objective procedures. Some have small sample sizes and others have quite large samples. Some health studies use animals as surrogates and others use human subjects. The following diagram does a great job of summarizing the different study types and the reliability of the results.

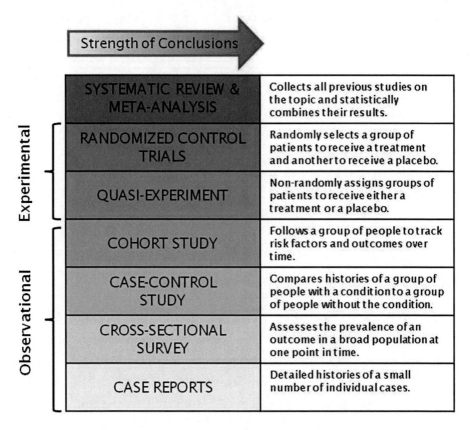

Figure 56 Study Types and Their Reliability.[173]

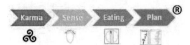

The Research Conflicts

At one time, hormone replacement was the therapy (HRT) of choice to reduce cancer, osteoporosis, and heart disease in women. Now HRT is considered harmful.[174]

The Prostate Specific Antigen (PSA) test used to be the standard-bearer for early detection of prostate cancer. Now, not so much.[175]

Low-fat diets (i.e. high-carb diets) are either the key to optimal heart health or the bane of our high LDL/low HDL/high triglyceride existence.[176]

These examples make the scene from the 1973 movie *Sleeper*, in which Woody Allen's character wakes up from a deep sleep in the distant future, seem prescient.[177,178] In that scene, the character baffles doctors in the future because he believes smoking is bad for you. A concept that seems so outlandish, it's intended to be the joke that it is. But other misconceptions held by Woody and the people of his time apparently aren't so clear. For example, that wheat germ and Tiger's Milk (America's Original Nutrition Bar) are good for you.[179,180,181]

The Media Only Reports The Hype

Yes, new research sometimes conflicts with old. Sometimes it stays consistently inconclusive but we only hear about the parts that are headline-worthy. According to some research, Echinacea shortens the duration of the common cold and lessens its symptoms.[182] But plenty of studies say it is completely ineffective.[183] We rarely hear about those.

The Healthcare Industrial Complex Rears Its Ugly Head

I hate to always pick on the HIC but they started it. The evidence of this conspiracy is just too blatant. As I'm writing this, the Coca Cola

---

Company, purveyor of sugar water in many colors and flavors, has been exposed in a multimillion dollar effort to fund scientists who claim that excess calories aren't the cause of obesity; lack of exercise is.[184]

Conflicts of interest happens all the time. Marion Nestle attempts to keep track of this on her Food Politics blog.[185] It's not a simple task since very few research databases allow you to easily find industry-sponsored research. Despite the complexity, she finds at least five studies per month with conflicts of interest. And less than 5% of these ever result in findings contrary to the sponsor's interest.

Physicians Have the Same Problem with the Results that We Do

Unfortunately, at the point of healthcare delivery, the problems continue. We live in a country where insurance companies make health care decisions instead of patients in consultation with their doctor. Doctors have limited time to critically assess the mounds of research and consider how it applies to you specifically. The result can be cookie-cutter, assembly-line healthcare with limited respect for you as an individual.

You Are Not "N"

Even if the research weren't biased, we'd still have the problem of "N." If you look at the primary sources of any research the media screams about, you'll consistently see a reference such as "N=1700," or "N= 102," or "N=8." In these instances, "N" stands for the number of subjects participating in the study. So in a study on inflammatory risk factors with women who drink wine, N=2900 means there were 2900 women in the study.[186]

Why is this a problem? Unless you are one of the 2900 women in the study, this research might be totally irrelevant to you. Although scientists do everything they can to represent the average person

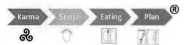

through randomized control trials, you are not an average person. No other person *ever* has your:

- Genetics
- Physiology
- Nutrition Habits
- Physical Activity Habits
- Mindset

None of the 2900 in "N" are the same as you. You're not even the same person you were when you first started reading this.

How to Apply this to *Your* Karma Sense Eating Plan

Does this mean we should ignore the research? No! When faced with the choice between anecdotes that say putting butter in my coffee will raise my IQ (as with so-called Bulletproof Coffee) and contradicting research that says it's more like Bullcrap coffee, I'll trust the research every time. Research is one of many factors we should consider when making healthcare decisions.

But when it comes to applying the constant swirl of wellness-related information from your doctor, friends, family, and the media, never forget that you are the expert on the subject of *YOU.* And while the research may scare you into a new health behavior, it does nothing to drive your long-term motivation. Long-term motivation must come from within.

This is a long way of saying that *The Karma Sense Eating Plan* is not prescriptive. It's realistic about all of these variables, and is designed to recognize that a one size fits all solution doesn't exist where health is concerned. Your mind and body are the best judges of a nutrition plan. There are people available to help you read the signals. But you are in charge. Because you are not "N."

In Closing...

Executive Summary

This section provides a few housekeeping details on items that may still pique your curiosity. They are:

- "I donate **all profits** from the sale of this book to charities that fight poverty and hunger." How does that work?
- What are next steps if I want to work with Davey H as my coach?

The Karma Sense Eating Plan and Charity

As part of *The Karma Sense Eating Plan*'s contribution to saving the world, I pledge to donate all profits from the sale of the book to charities that fight poverty and hunger. With that one simple promise, I open up a major can of worms (see mantra #2, Eat Protein in Every Meal). I'm the one who made that promise and even I'm asking:

- How do I define "profit?"
- How do I ensure that the profits are handled properly?
- How do I select these charities?

I want all readers to feel comfortable that I'm doing the right thing. I don't want you to worry about having a *Belle Gibson* situation. Belle Gibson is an Australian health blogger who made specious claims about her own health, promised that the proceeds of an app she created would go to charity, and then ran off with the money.[187]

In response, I'm taking all steps to provide as much transparency to the process as possible. I'll do this with two mechanisms.

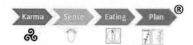

Provide Open Access to All Bookkeeping Associated with *The Karma Sense Eating Plan*

As of this writing, the only income associated with the book came from an Indiegogo crowdfunding campaign that helped kick start the project. Other anticipated income is from the actual sale of the book.

On the expense side, things are muddier. In some cases, especially early on, it's difficult to separate expenses that are investments in my coaching practice from pure book expenses. For example, Karma Sense™ is a registered trademark of my practice, Live Long Lead Long, LLC. There were significant expenses associated with that registration and it serves both the book and my practice.

To get around this, I only count the expenses that I can clearly trace to the production of the book. This includes things like editing and printing costs. By isolating these, it decreases the book's expenses and gets it to the charity-giving profit phase that much sooner.

Upon the book's release, I'll update my website quarterly with an accounting of its financials.

Create the Karma Sense Advisory Board to Provide Oversight

The Karma Sense Advisory Board serves as an independent steering committee. The board's current membership includes people who contributed to the crowd-sourcing campaign at a level that earned membership as a perk. In other words, they bought in.

At the time of this writing, the board consists of four people, including me. I'd welcome at least one more independent member. Board members names will be posted on my website once the book is released.

The board's charter is still in development. The mission is to donate as much money to charity as possible. Given that mission, responsibilities include, but are not limited to:

- Participate in all marketing decisions relating to *The Karma Sense Eating Plan* with the aim of maximizing sales without compromising the book's mission or putting undue stress on expenses.
- Monitor income and expenses associated with the creation and sale of *The Karma Sense Eating Plan* and provide good stewardship for all generated profits.
- Manage distribution of the profits generated from *The Karma Sense Eating Plan*. This includes selecting the target charities.

I want *The Karma Sense Eating Plan* to provide a mechanism to give back, to save the world. The above infrastructure ensures that this is the case.

How to Engage Davey H as a Coach

All kidding aside, the information and tools in *The Karma Sense Eating Plan* are designed to give you everything you need to be healthier, happier, and save the world on your terms and at your pace. Some people don't want to go it alone and for you, I sincerely hope you will consider me as a partner in your journey.

One reason I wrote *The Karma Sense Eating Plan* in the style that I did was to give you an idea of what it's like collaborating with me. I hope I demonstrated the following:

- I'm knowledgeable in the field of wellness.
- I keep my knowledge up-to-date.
- When pursuing a healthier you, I recognize that your needs and autonomy must be respected.
- I can discuss technical matters in an accessible way.
- I'll add a dash of fun to the process of being healthier, happier, and saving the world.

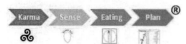

I know some people reading this won't appreciate my style and I view that as a victory for both of us. We won't waste each other's time trying to figure out if our chemistry is right.

If after reading this, you feel that I *can* help you in your journey to better health and happiness, here are some ways we can work together.

1. *Karma Sense Live* - a live presentation of *The Karma Sense Eating Plan*. The session lasts 90 minutes and includes audience participation. It provides a great opportunity to move your group, community, club, or gang towards better health and happiness.

2. *Karma Sense Mini Plan* - a two session coaching plan that includes a ninety minute introductory consultation, delivery of a plan for better health and happiness, a forty-five minute follow up session three to six weeks following the initial consultation, and electronic question and answer via email between the two sessions. Sessions occur either face-to-face or by telephone. If you want to pursue better health and happiness and don't want to commit to a partner in crime, this package is meant for you.

3. *Karma Sense Complete Coaching* - an Integrative Health, Nutrition, and Burnout Prevention coaching program that includes a ninety minute introductory session followed by five (5) forty-five minute sessions that are usually spread out over three months. Sessions take place face-to-face or by telephone. If your health goals can benefit from additional support and accountability, sign up for this plan.

4. *Karma Sense Enhanced Coaching* - an extended version of the *Karma Sense Complete* package. It includes the introductory session followed by ten forty-five minute sessions. The *Enhanced* package

---

provides an opportunity to work on complex wellness projects at a reduced cost.

5. *Karma Sense Kitchen/Grocery Shopping Boot Camp* - a two day experience in which we focus on your kitchen and grocery shopping habits and reinvent them for optimal health. This is a fantastic way to get dedicated support in streamlining your life for optimal health and happiness.

If one or more of these appeal to you or if you have a better idea how to work together, contact me through my web page, Live Long Lead Long. I relish the opportunity to work with you.

And, I don't have to stop there. If there is sufficient acceptance of *The Karma Sense Eating Plan*, I have a vision of expanding the ways to engage. This includes extending its reach in subject matter (e.g., *The Karma Sense Activity/Exercise Plan*, a dedicated cookbook), audience (e.g., *Karma Sense for kids*), and media (e.g., *The Karma Sense* podcast, *The Karma Sense* app). But much like the vision you create when building a *Karma Sense Eating Plan*, I need to take small discrete steps to get there.

The Karma Sense Eating Plan is one small step for karma and one giant leap for karma-kind.

Stuff at End of a Book

Glossary

A-Hole Inflection Point

The crossover point when someone's continued not-so-nice acts lead to consistent distrust by others.

Aerobic Exercise

Exercise of low to high intensity that depends primarily on the body's intake of oxygen.

Anaerobic Exercise

Exercise of high intensity that depends on more immediate forms of energy in the body such as ATP or glycogen.

Avoidable

A habit you'd like to keep or avoid but are flexible about or open to change.

Big Bang

Adopting all components of *The Karma Sense Eating Plan* in one fell swoop.

Bullcrap

Incredible; lacking credibility.

Bulletproof Diet

A diet fad that includes drinking coffee whipped with grass-fed butter and medium-chain-triglycerides (MCTs) which, in the case of the Bulletproof Diet, is what charlatans call "Coconut Oil." Because the MCTs they want you to buy from them is nothing but coconut oil.

Calorie-Dense

Foods that are high in calories relative to weight.

Carb-olicious Protein

A protein source that is relatively high in carbohydrates (e.g., beans).

Compliance

When you conform to the aspects of *The Karma Sense Eating Plan* that you selected.

Component

One of the four building blocks of *The Karma Sense Eating Plan*. These are the Karma, Sense, Eating, and Plan.

Constraint

Habits that you must continue (non-negotiable), prefer to continue (avoidable) or are a unique part of your identity (foible).

Conventional

(1) As it applies to growing food or practicing medicine, performing that activity in an unnatural and not always sensible way. (2) As it applies to everything else, the natural and sensible way of doing things.

Cruciferous Vegetable	Edible parts of plants in the cabbage family. Examples include broccoli and cabbage. These vegetables tend towards high nutrient density and low calories.
Doing Nothing	What most people call mindfulness.
Elimination Diets	Nutrition plans in which major food groups are avoided in order to drive calorie restriction. Gluten-free diets, Paleo diets, and raw food diets are all examples of elimination diets.
Embedded Constraint	A non-negotiable habit that is contrary to the guidelines of *The Karma Sense Eating Plan* but is inextricably tied to you. Embedded constraints are usually habits you are unable to give up as opposed to unwilling to give it up.
Fat-tastic Protein	A protein source that is relatively high in fat (e.g., nuts).
Feh!	A geezer's way of saying "I don't understand, but I want to express general disapproval anyway
Fell Swoop	Something to do with Shakespeare but nobody really knows. For the purposes of *The Karma Sense Eating Plan* a single fell swoop is the same as all at once.
Fer Shizzle	How cool kids said "for sure" in the 1990s
Foible	Your totally weird beliefs or habits that impact how and what you eat.
FUD	Fear, uncertainty, and doubt.
Happiness Catalyst	One of the many habits and actions that lead to greater happiness such as reading or recalling something for which you are grateful.
Healthcare Industrial Complex (HIC)	A giant consortium of public institutions, private companies, and so-called "not-for-profit" entities that appear to want to make you healthy and happy but, in fact, are motivated to keep you sick and depressed.
Healthy Lifestyle Militia (The Militia)	A smaller but still powerful counterforce to the HIC. The Militia takes extreme positions that are contrary to the "prevailing wisdom" espoused by the HIC. Many members of The Militia are sincere in their attempts to discover and distribute valuable information about wellness, but this group also contains members whose motivation is purely selfish.

High Intensity Interval Training (HIIT)	An exercise strategy alternating short periods of intense anaerobic exercise with less-intense recovery periods.
(Karma) Sensible Revolutionaries	A loose-knit rag-tag bunch who look out for our best interests and strive for moderation over extremism.
Kismet	An event that occurs as an act of fate or destiny. The lazy man's karma.
KSEP	Acronym for *The Karma Sense Eating Plan.*
Mantras	The five habits that are part of the Eating component.
Mind-FUL	Performing an action with intention and focus.
Mind-LESS	Performing an action in a careless, inattentive way; the things we usually do out of habit.
"N"	The number of subjects in a research study. Something that you usually are not.
Noncompliance	Times when you choose not to conform to the aspects of *The Karma Sense Eating Plan* that you selected.
Non-negotiable	Habits you choose not to give up.
Nutrient-dense	Foods that are high in macronutrients, micronutrients, and phytonutrients relative to their calorie content.
Origin Story	In comic book terminology, an account or back-story revealing how a character or team gained superpowers and/or the circumstances under which they became superheroes or supervillains.
Partial Adoption Approach	Taking on a subset of *The Karma Sense Eating Plan* components regardless of whether there is the intention to adopt the whole plan later.
Plan, The	A shorter term used to represent *The Karma Sense Eating Plan.*
Pre-Meal Ritual	The intentional and conscious acknowledgement of good deeds performed to honor the Karma component, gratitude for something someone did for you, and gratitude for the meal. The pre-meal ritual honors the Sense component.

Reducetarian	A person who eats less meat. Sometimes called a flexitarian.
Resistance Exercise	Exercise that focuses on applying an opposing force to natural muscle movement to induce muscular contraction which builds the strength, anaerobic endurance, and size of skeletal muscles. Weightlifting, for example.
Rickrolled	An Internet meme involving the music video for the 1987 Rick Astley song "Never Gonna Give You Up." The meme is a bait and switch; a person provides a hyperlink that is seemingly relevant to the topic at hand, but actually leads to Astley's video.
Save the World Model	Your personal view of how a better life would look. The model accepts that a saved world will consist of health and happiness for one or more of the following constituencies: • You • Your Loved Ones • The Population At Large • Other Sentient Beings • The Planet The model recognizes that people place different levels of priority to the constituencies listed.
Sexy-Time	Doing *it*.
Simple Equation	Calories consumed minus calories burned determines whether you lose weight (a negative result to the equation), maintain weight (the equation result equals zero), you gain weight (a positive result to the equation). The simple equation is where a person has the biggest influence on weight loss.
SMART Goal	A goal that is **S**pecific, **M**easurable, **A**chievable, **R**elevant and **T**ime-Bound.
Starchy Vegetable	The edible part of a plant that is high in complex carbohydrates.
Steady State Exercise	Activity that achieves a balance between the energy requi red by working muscles and the rate of oxygen and delive ry for aerobic ATP production. Exercising at a near constant speed usually for a sustained period of time.

| Tasty-But-Empty-Calorie Cabal | A full dues paying member of the HIC. The cabal manufactures two kinds of foods. They market the first as healthy but it's not. The second kind has no healthy pretense but is specifically engineered for you to crave. Amazingly, both kinds of foods are often sold by the same companies. |
| Zone of Trust and Support | The cushion of acceptance that is given to people who are good and nice. |

The Karma Sense Eating Plan

Notes

Executive Summary (Introduction)

[1] Fast Company Staff. "The World's Top 10 Most Innovative Companies of 2015 in Fitness." *Fast Company*, February 10, 2015. Accessed September 30, 2015. http://www.fastcompany.com/3041643/most-innovative-companies-2015/the-worlds-top-10-most-innovative-companies-of-2015-in-fitnes.

[2] "Best Medical Schools: Research." *U.S. News and World Report Education*, 2015. Accessed September 30, 2015. http://grad-schools.usnews.rankingsandreviews.com/best-graduate-schools/top-medical-schools/research-rankings?int=af3309&int=b3b50a&int=b14409.

[3] Schatzker, Mark. *The Dorito Effect*. New York: Simon & Schuster, 2015.

[4] Schatzker, The *Dorito Effect*.

[5] "GDP by Industry/VA, GO, II." *Gross Domestic Product (GDP) By Industry Data*. Bureau of Economic Analysis. U.S. Department of Commerce. (2014). http://www.bea.gov/industry/xls/io-annual/GDPbyInd_VA_NAICS_1997-2014.xlsx.

[6] *Close Encounters of the Third Kind*. Directed by Steven Spielberg. Culver City, CA: Columbia Pictures. 1977.

[7] Photo Credit: mptvimages.com

[8] "Carl Douglas – Kung fu fighting (original)." Video, 03:09. *YouTube*. Posted March 2008. https://www.youtube.com/watch?v=jhUkGIsKvn0.

[9] Guevarra, Darwin A., and Ryan T. Howell. "To have in order to do: Exploring the effects of consuming experiential products on well-being." Journal of Consumer Psychology 25, no. 1 (2015): 28-41. doi:10.1016/j.jcps.2014.06.006.

Navigating The Karma Sense Eating Plan

[10] *Rick Astley Never Gonna Give You Up* 7 Inch Single Cover. Wikimedia Foundation. March 5, 2008. Accessed September 17, 2015. https://en.wikipedia.org/wiki/File:RickAstleyNeverGonnaGiveYouUp7InchSingleCover.jpg

[11] This image is provided as satire. It is of sufficient resolution for commentary and identification but lower resolution than the original cover. Copies made from it will be of inferior quality, unsuitable as artwork on pirate versions or other uses that would compete with the commercial purpose of the original artwork.

The Karma Sense Eating Plan Origin Story

[12] Bennett, Mary P., Janice M. Zeller, Lisa Rosenberg, and Judith McCann. "The Effect of Mirthful Laughter on Stress and Natural Killer Cell Activity." *Alternative Therapies in Health and Medicine* 9, no. 2 (2013): 38-45. http://www.ncbi.nlm.nih.gov/pubmed/12652882.

[13] Lund, Dale A., Rebecca L. Utz, Michael Caserta, Brian de Vries. "Humor, Laughter & Happiness in the Daily Lives of Recently Bereaved Spouses." *Omega* 58, no. 2 (2008): 87–105. http://www.ncbi.nlm.nih.gov/pmc/articles/PMC2646184/.

[14] Image credit: David Hellman

The Karma Sense Eating Plan Overview

[15] Oppenheimer, Todd. "The Vegetable Detective: A molecular biologist is finding what could be dangerous levels of heavy metals in plants like kale, often called the 'queen' of the vegetable kingdom. And they've shown up the most in organic varieties." *Craftsmanship.* July 7, 2015. Accessed July 26, 2015. http://craftsmanship.net/the-vegetable-detective/

[16] Hari, Vani. "Subway: Stop Using Dangerous Chemicals in Your Bread." *Food Babe.* Accessed July 26, 2015. http://foodbabe.com/subway/.

[17] "'Yoga Mat' Material Found in Nearly 500 Foods." *Environmental Working Group.* February 27, 2014. Accessed July 26, 2015. http://www.ewg.org/release/yoga-mat-chemical-found-nearly-500-foods.

[18] Weil, Andrew. "Wheat Belly Diet: Is Wheat Dangerous" *Weil.* February 19, 2013. Accessed July 26 2015. http://www.drweil.com/drw/u/QAA401243/Wheat-Belly-Diet-Is-Wheat-Dangerous.html.

[19] Gunnars, Kris. "3 Reasons Why Bulletproof Coffee is a Bad Idea." *Authority Nation.* June 2014. Accessed July 26, 2015. http://authoritynutrition.com/3-reasons-why-bulletproof-coffee-is-a-bad-idea/.

[20] This quote is often attributed to Leo Deroucher. According to multiple sources, including the infallible *Wikipedia*, he did not actually say that. He said, "The nice guys are all over there, in seventh place." However, after journalists condensed it to the better known saying, he took it on as his own.

[21] "Leo Durocher." *Wikipedia.* November 17, 2015. Accessed November 23, 2015. https://en.wikipedia.org/wiki/Leo_Durocher

[22] Image credit: David Hellman.

[23] Grant, Adam M. *Give and Take: Why Helping Others Drives Our Success*. New York: Viking. 2013.

[24] Image credit: David Hellman.

[25] Although this quote is liberally attributed to Ms. Johnson throughout the Twittersphere, I haven't found any reference to her actually saying it herself. I politely (really, I was polite and not stalker-y at all) reached out to Chalene Johnson on multiple occasions to seek confirmation that she actually said it. I never heard back. What did she teach?

[26] Ennis, Tyler. *Twitter*. November 7, 2015, 6:00 pm. https://twitter.com/myblocktyler/status/663128867285135360.

[27] *Bill & Ted's Excellent Adventure*. Directed by Stephen Hereck. 1989. Los Angeles: Orion Pictures.

[28] Photo Source: Creative Licensing Corporation.

[29] *Google Scholar*. Accessed July 27, 2015. https://scholar.google.com/scholar?hl=en&q=gratitude+happiness+research&btnG=&as_sdt=1%2C47&as_sdtp=.

Karma: The Best Way to Start Your Day

[30] Image credit: David Hellman.

[31] Jones, Damon E., Mark Greenberg, and Max Crowley. "Early Social-Emotional Functioning and Public Health: The Relationship Between Kindergarten Social Competence and Future Wellness." *American Journal of Public Health*. 105, no. 11 (2015): doi:10.2105/AJPH.2015.302630.

[32] Chatterjee, Arijit and Donald C. Hambrick. "It's All about Me: Narcissistic Chief Executive Officers and Their Effects on Company Strategy and Performance." *Administrative Science Quarterly*. 52, no. 3 (2007): 351-386. doi:10.2189/asqu.52.3.351.

[33] Thaler, Linda Kaplan, and Robin Koval. *The Power of Nice: How to Conquer the Business World with Kindness*. New York: Crown Business, 2006.

[34] Kashdan, Todd, and Robert Biswas-Diener. *The Upside of Your Dark Side: Why Being Your Whole Self – Not Just Your "Good" Self – Drives Success and Fulfillment*. New York: Hudson Street Press, 2014.

[35] *Google Scholar*. Accessed December 12, 2015. https://scholar.google.com/scholar?hl=en&q=personal+relationships+and+health&btnG=&as_sdt=1%2C47&as_sdtp=

[36] Image credit: David Hellman.

[37] Image credit: David Hellman.

[38] Image credit: David Hellman.

Common Sense + Sensitivity = Karma Sense
[39] Image credit: David Hellman.

[40] Photo credit: iStockphoto; powerofforever.

[41] *Pee-wee's Big Adventure*. Directed by Tim Burton. 1985. Burbank, CA: Warner Bros.

[42] Photo credit: Warner Bros. Studios. Used for satirical purposes.

Sense: Shake It Up Break It Down
[43] Photo credit: Amazon.com, Inc.

[44] Ocasek, Ric. "Shake It Up." MP3. Elektra Records. 1981.

[45] Swift, Taylor and Max Martin-Shellback. "Shake It Off." MP3. Big Machine Records. 2014.

[46] Gomez, Selena. "Shake It Up." MP3. Walt Disney Records. 2011.

[47] Robinson, Eric, Paul Aveyard, Amanda Daley, Kate Jolly, Amanda Lewis, Deborah Lycett, and Suzanne Higgs. "Eating attentively: a systematic review and meta-analysis of the effect of food intake memory and awareness on eating." *The American Journal of Clinical Nutrition* 97, no. 4 (2013): 728-742. doi:10.3945/acjn.112.045245.

[48] Dalen, Jeanne, Bruce W. Smith, Brian M. Shelley, Anita Lee Sloan, Lisa Leahigh, and Debbie Begay. "Pilot study: Mindful Eating and Living (MEAL): Weight, eating behavior, and psychological outcomes associated with a mindfulness-based intervention for people with obesity." *Complementary Therapies in Medicine*. 18, no. 6 (2010): 260-264. http://www.complementarytherapiesinmedicine.com/article/S0965-2299(10)00104-4/abstract.

[49] Emmons, Robert A., and Michael E. McCullough. "Counting blessings versus burdens: An experimental investigation of gratitude and subjective well-being in daily life." *Journal of Personality and Social Psychology*. 84, no. 2 (2003): 377-389. http://psycnet.apa.org/journals/psp/84/2/377/.

[50] Achor, Shawn. "The Happiness Advantage: Linking Positive Brains to Performance." *TEDx Talks*. Video 12:20. YouTube Filmed May 2011. Posted June 2011. https://www.youtube.com/watch?v=GXy__kBVq1M.

[51] Photo credit: iStockphoto; RapidEye.

52 Image credit: David Hellman.

53 Image credit: David Hellman.

A Quick Reintroduction to the *Eating* Component

54 Image credit: David Hellman.

55 Mata, Jutta, Peter M. Todd, and Sonia Lippke. "When weight management lasts. Lower perceived rule complexity increases adherence." *Appetite*. 54, no. 1 (2010): 37-43 doi:10.1016/j.appet.2009.09.004.

56 Murray, Ed. *A tower and museum honoring Thomas Edison sit on 34 acres of land in the Middlesex County town named after the famed inventor. The museum officially re-opens this weekend after a renovation.* New Jersey Online, Newark. June 10, 2012.

57 "The Doctor of the Future." *Snopes.com: Rumor Has It*. January 25, 2015. Accessed August 3, 2015. http://www.snopes.com/quotes/futuredoctor.asp.

58 Adams, Kelly M., Martin Kohlmeier, and Stephen H. Zeisel. "Nutrition Education in U.S. Medical Schools: Latest Update of a National Survey." *Academic Medicine*. 85, no. 9 (2010): 1537-1542. doi:10.1097/ACM.0b013e3181eab71b.

Mantra #1: Eat Slowly and Stop Before You're Full

59 "Choose MyPlate.Gov: About Us." *United States Department of Agriculture*. June 2, 2011. Accessed August 2, 2015. http://www.choosemyplate.gov/about-us.

60 "MyPyramid." *Wikipedia*. May 14, 2015. Accessed August 2, 2015. https://en.wikipedia.org/wiki/MyPyramid.

61 Image credit: "MyPyramidFood" by United States Department of Agriculture - http://www.mypyramid.gov. Licensed under Public Domain via Commons - https://commons.wikimedia.org/wiki/File:MyPyramidFood.svg#/media/File:MyPyramidFood.svg.

62 "Eat Slow, Lose Weight?" *WebMD: Diet and Management*. November 17, 2004. Accessed August 2, 2015. http://www.webmd.com/diet/20041117/eat-slow-lose-weight.

63 Young, Lisa R. and Marion Nestle. "The Contribution of Expanding Portion Sizes to the US Obesity Epidemic." *American Journal of Public Health*. 92, no. 2 (2002): 246-249. Accessed August 2, 2015. http://www.ncbi.nlm.nih.gov/pmc/articles/PMC1447051/.

64 Kreuter, M. W., S. G. Chheeda, and F. C. Bull. "How does physician advice influence patient behavior? Evidence for a priming effect." *Archives of Family Medicine.* 9, no. 5 (2000): 426-433.
http://www.ncbi.nlm.nih.gov/pubmed/10810947

65 "Waist Size Matters." *Harvard T. H. Chan School of Public Health.* Accessed December 6, 2015. http://www.hsph.harvard.edu/obesity-prevention-source/obesity-definition/abdominal-obesity/.

Mantra #2: Eat Protein in Every Meal

66 *Fast Times at Ridgemont High.* Directed by Amy Heckerling. 1982. Universal City, CA: Universal Pictures.

67 Photo Credit: Courtesy of Universal Studios Licensing LLC. ©1982 Universal City Studios, Inc.

68 Photo Credit: Abraham Hellman.

69 Photo Credit: Glen Hellman

70 Atkins, Robert C. *Dr. Atkins' Diet Revolution: The High Calorie Way to Stay Thin Forever.* Philadelphia: D. McKay Co. 1972.

71 Price, Roger, and Leonard Stern. *Star Wars Mad Libs.* Los Angeles: Price Stern Sloan. 2008.

72 Image credit: David Hellman.

73 Nierenberg, Cari. "How Much Protein Do You Need?" *WebMD.* February 28, 2011. Accessed August 25, 2015. http://www.webmd.com/diet/healthy-kitchen-11/how-much-protein.

74 Photo credit: iStockphoto; inarik, Yasonya. Modified by David Hellman.

75 Hellman, David. *Live Long Lead Long.* Accessed November 30, 2015. http://www.livelongleadlong.com/?s=healthcare+industrial+complex.

76 Poortmans, J. R., and O. Dellalieux. "Do regular high protein diets have potential health risks on kidney functions in athletes?" *Journal of the International Society of Sports Nutrition.* 10, no. 1 (2000): 28-38.
http://www.ncbi.nlm.nih.gov/pubmed/10722779.

77 Kerstetler, J. E., A. M. Kenney, and K. L. Insogna. "Dietary protein and skeletal health: a review of recent human research." *Current Opinion in Lipidology.* 22, no. 1 (2011). 16-20. doi:10.1097/MOL.0b013e3283419441.

78 Gannon, Mary C., and Frank Q. Nuttal. "Effect of High-Protein, Low-Carbohydrate Diet on Blood Glucose Control In People With Type 2 Diabetes."

Diabetes. 53, no. 9 (2004): 2375-2382.
http://diabetes.diabetesjournals.org/content/53/9/2375.full.pdf.

[79] Moyer, Melinda W., and Dean Ornish. "Why Almost Everything Dean Ornish Says About Nutrition is Wrong. UPDATED: With Dean Ornish's Response." *Scientific American*, June 1, 2015. Accessed August, 2, 2015. http://www.scientificamerican.com/article/why-almost-everything-dean-ornish-says-about-nutrition-is-wrong/.

[80] Nodolsky, Spencer. "High-Protein Diets Linked to Cancer: Should You Be Concerned?" *Examine.com*. March 6, 2014. Accessed August 3, 2015. http://examine.com/blog/high-protein-diets-linked-to-cancer-should-you-be-concerned/.

[81] Sisson, Mark. "Dear Mark: Does Eating a Low Carb Diet Cause Insulin Resistance?" *Mark's Daily Apple*. August 27, 2012. Accessed August 2, 2015. http://www.marksdailyapple.com/does-eating-low-carb-cause-insulin-resistance/#axzz3sMnFKbQQ.

[82] "Position of the American Dietetic Association: Vegetarian Diets." *Journal of the American Dietetic Association*. 109. (2009): 1266-1282. Accessed August 2, 2015. http://www.vrg.org/nutrition/2009_ADA_position_paper.pdf.

[83] Shah, Meena, Vinaya Simha, and Abhimanyu Garg. "Long-Term Impact of Bariatric Surgery on Body Weight, Comorbidities, and Nutritional Status." *The Journal of Clinical Endocrinology & Metabolism*. 91, no. 11 (2013): doi:10.1210/jc.2006-0557.

[84] MacLean, Lloyd D., Barbara M. Rhode, and Carl W. Nohr. "Late Outcome of Isolated Gastric Bypass." *Annals of Surgery*. 231, no. 4 (2000): 524-528. http://www.ncbi.nlm.nih.gov/pmc/articles/PMC1421028/.

Mantra #3: Eat More Vegetables and Fruits

[85] Photo Credit: Unknown Professional Bar Mitzah Photographer.

[86] Mauer, Lilli, Ahmed El-Sohemey. "Prevalence of cilantro (Coriandrum sativum) disliking among different ethnocultural groups." *Flavour*. 1, no. 8 (2012): 1-7. doi:10.1186/2044-7248-1-8.

[87] "Supertasters." *Wikipedia*. October 25, 2015 Accessed December 15, 2015. https://en.wikipedia.org/wiki/Supertaster

[88] Mennella, Julie A., Coren P. Jagnow, and Gary K. Beauchamp. "Prenatal and Postnatal Flavor Learning by Human Infants." *Pediatrics*. 107, no. 6 (2001): 1-6. 2001. http://pediatrics.aappublications.org/content/107/6/e88.short.

[89] Hellman, David, "The Worst Advice Ever? Unsolicited!" *Live Long Lead Long* (blog), April 26, 2015. http://www.livelongleadlong.com/coaching-methodology/readiness-to-change/unsolicited-advice-and-why-it-doesnt-work/.

[90] Hellman, David, "How Isaac Newton's Health Coach Helped Him Discover His Three Laws of Motion." *Live Long Lead Long* (blog), April 29, 2015. http://www.livelongleadlong.com/coaching-methodology/readiness-to-change/isaac-newtons-health-coach-and-three-laws-of-motion/.

[91] "Beaver Won't Eat." Video, 03:10. *YouTube*. Circa 1957-1963. Posted October 2011. https://www.youtube.com/watch?v=0SFSGTdaulc.

[92] Photo Credit: Courtesy of Universal Studios Licensing LLC. ©1982 Universal City Studios, Inc.

[93] "AICR's Foods That Fight Cancer: Broccoli and Cruciferous Vegetables." *American Institute for Cancer Research*. May 14, 2014. Accessed August 3, 2014. http://www.aicr.org/foods-that-fight-cancer/broccoli-cruciferous.html.

[94] Lund University. "Spinach extract decreases cravings, aids weight loss." *ScienceDaily*. September 2, 2014. Accessed August 3, 2015. http://www.sciencedaily.com/releases/2014/09/140902114928.htm.

[95] Gao, Xiangqun , Albena T. Dinkova-Kostova, and Paul Talalay. "Powerful and prolonged protection of human retinal pigment epithelial cells, keratinocytes, and mouse leukemia cells against oxidative damage: The indirect antioxidant effects of sulforaphane." *Proceedings of the National Academy of Sciences of the United States of America*. 98, no. 26 (2001): 15221-15226. 2001. doi:10.1073/pnas.261572998.

[96] White, Bonnie A., Caroline C. Horwath, and Tamlin S. Conner. "Many apples a day keep the blues away – Daily experiences of negative and positive affect and food consumption in young adults." *British Journal of Health Psychology*. 18, no. 4 (2013): 782–798. doi:10.1111/bjhp.12021.

[97] Karakula, H., A. Opolska, A, Kowal, M. Domański, A. Plotka, and J. Perzyński. "Does diet affect our mood? The significance of folic acid and homocysteine." *Polski Merkuriusz Lekarski*. 26, no. 152 (2009): 136-141. http://www.ncbi.nlm.nih.gov/pubmed/19388520.

[98] Jacka Felice N., Simon Overland, Robert Stewart, Grethe S. Tell, Ingvar Bjelland, and Arnstein Mykletun. "Association Between Magnesium Intake and Depression and Anxiety in Community-Dwelling Adults: The Hordaland Health Study" *Australian and New Zealand Journal of Psychiatry*. 43, no. 1 (2009): 45-52. doi:10.1080/00048670802534408.

[99] Gomez-Pinilla, Fernando, and Trang T. J, Nguyen. "Natural mood foods: The actions of polyphenols against psychiatric and cognitive disorders." *Nutritional Neuroscience.* 15, no. 3 (2012): 127-133. May 2012 Accessed August 3, 2015. doi:10.1179/1476830511Y.0000000035.

[100] Image credit: David Hellman

[101] Jacobellis v. Ohio, Ohio St. 22, 179 N.E.2d 777 (1964). Accessed November 24, 2015. https://www.law.cornell.edu/supremecourt/text/378/184.

[102] Giller, Chip. "The Way I See It." Starbucks Coffee Cup. Starbucks Corporation. #289. 2006.

[103] Fitzgerald, F. Scott. "The Crack-Up." *Esquire*, Winter 1936. Published online February 26, 2008. Accessed November 24, 2015. http://www.esquire.com/news-politics/a4310/the-crack-up/.

[104] "Meat Eater's Guide: Climate and Environmental Impacts." *Environmental Working Group.* 2011. Accessed August 4, 2015. http://www.ewg.org/meateatersguide/a-meat-eaters-guide-to-climate-change-health-what-you-eat-matters/climate-and-environmental-impacts/.

[105] Photo credit: Evan Amos, Wikipedia.

[106] Photo credit: David Hellman

[107] Osman, Larry. *Put It In Your Act!* Bridgewater, NJ: Lulu. 2009.

Mantra #4: Eat Whole Food Carbohydrates After Vigorous Exercise

[108] Adapted from *Adam and Eve in the Garden of Eden.* Origina by Lucas Cranach. 1531. Adaptation by David Hellman.

[109] "Kellogg's Corn Flakes with Superman and Jimmy Olsen." Video, 00:58. *YouTube* Circa 1952-1958. Posted February 2009. https://www.youtube.com/watch?v=pPwgG2wNn3Y&feature=youtu.be.

[110] Photo credit: YouTube. Photo used for instructional purposes related to commentary on changing standards in broadcasting content.

[111] "Adventures of Superman Trivia. *IMDb.* Accessed December 16, 2015. http://www.imdb.com/title/tt0044231/trivia.

[112] Levine, Deborah J. *Lois and Clark.* Directed by Deborah J. Levine. 1993-1997. American Broadcasting Company.

[113] Photo credit: American Broadcasting Company. Photo used for instructional purposes related to commentary on changing standards in broadcasting content.

[114] *Monty Python and the Holy Grail.* Directed by Terry Gilliam and Terry Jones. London: EMI Films. 1975.

[115] Image credit: David Hellman.

[116] "Measuring Physical Activity Intensity." *Centers for Disease Control and Prevention, Division of Nutrition, Physical Activity, and Obesity.* June 4, 2015. Accessed August 8, 2015. http://www.cdc.gov/physicalactivity/basics/measuring/.

[117] Clift, Stephen, Grenville Hancox, Ian Morrison, Bärbel Hess, Gunter Kreutz, and Don Stewart. "Choral singing and psychological wellbeing: Findings from English choirs in a crossnational survey using the WHOQOL-BREF." *International Symposium on Performance Science.* 2007. http://www98.griffith.edu.au/dspace/bitstream/handle/10072/17825/48495_1?sequence=1.

[118] Baker, Felicity, and T. Wigram. "The immediate and long term effects of singing on the mood states of people with Traumatic Brain injury." *British Journal of Music Therapy* 18, no. 2 (2004): 55-64. http://espace.library.uq.edu.au/view/UQ:74062.

[119] Cohen, Mary L. "Choral singing and prison inmates: Influences of performing in a prison choir." *Journal of Correctional Education* 60, no. 1 March (2009): 52-65. http://www.jstor.org/stable/23282774.

[120]Shulman, Max. *The Many Loves of Dobie Gillis* Directed by Rod Amateau, et. al. 1959-1963. Columbia Broadcasting System.

[121] Photo credit: Unknown. Photo used for satirical purposes only.

[122] Mathieson, R. A., J. L. Walberg, F. C. Gwazdauskas, D. E. Hinkle. and J. M. Gregg. "The effect of varying carbohydrate content of a very-low-caloric diet on resting metabolic rate and thyroid hormones." *Metabolism.* 35, no. 5 (1986): 394-398. http://www.ncbi.nlm.nih.gov/pubmed/3702673.

[123] Anderson, K. E., W. Rosner, M. S. Khan, M. I. New, S. Y. Pang, P. S. Wissel, and A. Kappas. "Diet-hormone interactions: protein/carbohydrate ratio alters reciprocally the plasma levels of testosterone and cortisol and their respective binding globulins in man." *Life Sciences,* 40, no. 18 (1987): 1761-1768. http://www.ncbi.nlm.nih.gov/pubmed/3573976.

[124] Mehler, Philip S. and Mori Krantz. "Anorexia Nervosa Medical Issues." *Journal of Women's Health.* 12, no. 4 (2003): 331-340. doi:10.1089/154099903765448844.

[125] Lane, A. R., J. W. Duke, and A. C. Hackney. "Influence of dietary carbohydrate intake on the free testosterone: cortisol ratio responses to short-term intensive exercise training." *European Journal of Applied Physiology.* 108, no. 6 (2010): 1125-1131. http://link.springer.com/article/10.1007%2Fs00421-009-1220-5.

[126] Wood, Joanne V., Elaine W. Q. Perunovic, and John W. Lee. "Positive Self-Statements. Power for Some, Peril for Others." *Pyschological Science.* 20, no. 7 (2009): 860-866. doi:10.1111/j.1467-9280.2009.02370.x.

[127] Feibusch, Joshua M., Peter R. Holt. "Impaired absorptive capacity for carbohydrate in the aging human." *Digestive Diseases and Sciences.* 27, no. 12 (1982): 1095-1100. http://link.springer.com/article/10.1007/BF01391447.

Mantra #5: Eat Good Fats Daily and Balance a Variety of Good Fats

[128] Roddenberry, Gene. *Star Trek.* Directed by Gene Roddenberry. 1966-1969. National Broadcasting Company. 1966-1969.

[129] Photo credit: Columbia Broadcasting System. Photo used for satirical purposes.

[130] Gardner, Bruce L. *American Agriculture in the Twentieth Century.* Cambridge, MA: Harvard University Press. 2002.

[131] Katz, David. "Scapegoats, Saints and Saturated Fats: Old Mistakes in New Directions." *Huffpost Healthy Living.* October 24, 2014. Accessed August 9, 2015. http://www.huffingtonpost.com/david-katz-md/saturated-fat_b_4156320.html.

[132] "SnackWell's." SnackWell's. Back to Nature Foods Company, LLC. Product Package. August 9, 2015.

[133] "Dietary Guidelines." *Office of Disease Prevention and Health Promotion.* August 9, 2015. Accessed August 9, 2015. http://health.gov/dietaryguidelines/.

[134] "New evidence raises questions about the link between fatty acids and heart disease." *News: Research.* University of Cambridge. March 18, 2014. Accessed August 9, 2015. http://www.cam.ac.uk/research/news/new-evidence-raises-questions-about-the-link-between-fatty-acids-and-heart-disease.

[135] "Chocolate Peanut Butter Bar." Atkins Bars. Atkins Nutritionals. Product Package. August 9, 2015.

[136] "Chia Shrek Handmade Decorative Planter." *Amazon*. Accessed August 9, 2015. http://www.amazon.com/Chia-Handmade-Decorative-Discontinued-Manufacturer/dp/B000AIGBFA/ref=sr_1_1?ie=UTF8&qid=1448375945&sr=8-1&keywords=chia+shrek.

[137] "Trans Fats." *Nutrition for Everyone: Basics*. Centers for Disease Control and Prevention. Accessed 9, 2015. http://www.cdc.gov/nutrition/images/nutrition-label.gif.

Playing With *The Karma Sense Eating Plan*

[138] "Pirates (Faction)." *Wikia: Brickapedia*. Accessed August 9, 2015. http://lego.wikia.com/wiki/Pirates_(Faction).

[139] Image credit: David Hellman.

[140] Simon, Paul. "50 Ways to Leave Your Lover." MP3. Columbia Records. 1975.

[141] Caldwell, Karen L., Jennifer Gray, and Ruth Q. Wolever. "The Process of Patient Empowerment in Integrative Health Coaching: How Does it Happen?" *Global Advances in Health and Medicine*. 2, no. 3 (2013): 48-57. http://www.gahmj.com/doi/abs/10.7453/gahmj.2013.026.

[142] Image credit: David Hellman.

[143] Berra, Yogi and Dave Kaplan. *When You Come to a Fork in the Road, Take It!: Inspiration and Wisdom From One of Baseball's Greatest Heroes*. Hyperion: New York, 2001.

[144] *Pee-wee's Big Adventure*. Directed by Tim Burton. 1985. Burbank, CA: Warner Bros.

[145] Photo credit: Warner Brothers Studios. Photo used for satirical purposes.

[146] "Mighty Morphin Power Rangers Legacy Dino Megazord Action Figure." *GeekAlerts: Gadgets for Geeks*. January 17, 2015. Accessed August 10, 2015. http://www.geekalerts.com/mighty-morphin-power-rangers-legacy-dino-megazord-action-figure/.

[147] "Mighty Morphin' Power Rangers Morph [HQ]." Video , 01:45. *YouTube*. Posted October 16, 2006. https://www.youtube.com/watch?v=C1UtsY0uZVk.

[148] Moore, Latitia V. and Frances E. Thompson. "Adults Meeting Fruit and Vegetable Intake Recommendations — United States, 2013." *Morbidity and Mortality Weekly Report.* 64, no. 26 (2015): 709-713. http://www.cdc.gov/mmwr/preview/mmwrhtml/mm6426a1.htm.

[149] Gripetag, Lena, Jarl Torgerson, Jan Karlsson, and Anna K. Lindroos. "Prolonged refeeding improves weight maintenance after weight loss with very-low energy diets." *British Journal of Nutrition.* 103, no. 01 (2010): 141-148. doi:10.1017/S0007114509991474.

[150] Coelho do Vale, Rita and Marcel Zeelenberg Rik Pieters. "The Benefits of Behaving Badly on Occasion: Successful Regulation by Planned Hedonic Deviations." *Advances in Consumer Research.* 42 (2014): 437-438. http://www.journals.elsevier.com/journal-of-consumer-psychology/forthcoming-articles/the-benefits-of-behaving-badly-on-occasion-successful/.

[151] Milne, A. A., "Chapter X. In Which Christopher Robin Give Pooh a Party, and We Say Good-bye." *Winnie the Pooh.* 160. New York: E. P. Dutton & Co., Inc. 1954.

Food Lists

[152] "Cruciferous Vegetables." *Wikipedia.* April 8, 2015. Accessed August 4, 2015. https://en.wikipedia.org/wiki/Cruciferous_vegetables.

[153] "Starchy Vegetables." *MDhealth.com.* Accessed August 4, 2015. http://www.md-health.com/Starchy-Vegetables.html.

[154] Hobson, Katherine. "11 Best Fish: High in Omega 3s – and Environmentally-Friendly." *U.S. News & World Report.* May 29, 2009. Accessed August 9, 2015. http://health.usnews.com/health-news/diet-fitness/slideshows/best-fish.

[155] "National Nutrition Database for Standard Reference Release 27." *Agricultural Research Service.* United States Department of Agriculture. Accessed August 15, 2015. http://ndb.nal.usda.gov/ndb/foods.

[156] "Nutrient Search." *SELF Nutrition Data.* 2014. Accessed August 15, 2015. http://nutritiondata.self.com/tools/nutrient-search.

Karma Sense Cooking

[157] Wolfson, Julia A. and Sara N. Bleich, "Is cooking at home associated with better diet quality or weight loss intention?" *Public Health Nutrition.* 18, no. 8 (2015): 1397-1406. doi:10.1017/S1368980014001943.

[158] An, R. "Fast-food and full-service restaurant consumption and daily energy and nutrient intakes in US adults." *European Journal of Clinical Nutrition*. July 1, 2015. doi:10.1038/ejcn.2015.104.

[159] "Calories burned in 30 minutes for people of three different weights." *Harvard Health Publications*. Harvard Medical School. July 1, 2004. Accessed 16, 2015. http://www.health.harvard.edu/diet-and-weight-loss/calories-burned-in-30-minutes-of-leisure-and-routine-activities.

[160] Photo credit: Marcus Embry.

[161] dae18 "Oopsie Bread." *Food.com*. Accessed November 24, 2015. http://www.food.com/recipe/oopsie-bread-497736.

Plan Tools

[162] Miller, William R, and Stephen Rollnick. "Exploring Values and Goals." *Motivational Interviewing*. New York: Guilford Press. 2013 80-83.

Super Wowie Bonus Fun

[163] Theobald, H., L. O. Bygren, J. Carstensen, and P. Engfeldt. "A Moderate Intake of Wine is Associated with Reduced Total Mortality and Reduced Mortality from Cardiovascular Disease." *Journal of Studies on Alcohol*. 61, no. 5 (2000): 652-656. doi:10.15288/jsa.2000.61.652.

[164] *There's Something About Mary*. Directed Bobby Farrelly and Peter Farrelly. 1988. Los Angeles: Twentieth Century Fox Film Corporation.

[165] "ACSM Issues New Recommendations on Quantity and Quality of Exercise." *News Releases*. American College of Sports Medicine. Accessed August 13, 2015. http://www.acsm.org/about-acsm/media-room/news-releases/2011/08/01/acsm-issues-new-recommendations-on-quantity-and-quality-of-exercise.

[166] "2008 Physical Guidelines for Americans Summary." *Office of Disease Prevention and Health Promotion*. 2008. Accessed August 13, 2015. http://health.gov/paguidelines/guidelines/summary.aspx.

[167] Bouchez, Colette. "How Much Exercise Do You Really Need?" *WebMD: Fitness & Exercise*. June24, 2010. Accessed September 15, 2015. http://www.webmd.com/fitness-exercise/getting-enough-exercise.

[168] Tabata, Izumi, Kouji Nishimura, Motoki Kouzaki, Yuusuke Hirai, Futoshi Ogita, Motohiko Miyachi, and Kaoru Yamamoto. "Effects of moderate-intensity endurance and high-intensity intermittent training on anaerobic capacity and VO2max." *Medicine and Science in Sports and Exercise*. 28, no. 10 (1996): 1327-1330. http://journals.lww.com/acsm-

msse/pages/articleviewer.aspx?year=1996&issue=10000&article=00018&type=a
bstract.

[169] Tremblay, Angelo, Jean-Aimé Simoneau, and Claude Bouchard. "Impact of Exercise Intensity on Body Fatness and Skeletal Muscle Metabolism." *Metabolism*. 43, no. 7 (1994): 814-818. doi:10.1016/0026-0495(94)90259-3

[170] Zuhl, Michael and Len Kravitz. "HIIT vs. Continuous Endurance Training: Battle of the Aerobic Titans." *IDEA Fitness Journal*. 9, no. 2 (2012): 34-40. http://www.ideafit.com/fitness-library/hiit-vs-continuous-endurance-training-battle-of-the-aerobic-titans

[171] Ratliff, Bob. "Researcher advises: To save mall time, park and walk." *Mississippi State University*. April 1, 1998. Accessed April 18, 2015. http://www.msstate.edu/newsroom/article/1998/04/researcher-advises-save-mall-time-park-and-walk/.

[172] Hellman, David. "Healthy Transportation – The Mental Calculation.' *Live Long Lead Long* (blog), January 23, 2015. http://www.livelongleadlong.com/woh/movement-exercise-rest/personal-transportation-mental-calculation/.

[173] Belluz, Julia and Steven Hoffman. "The one chart you need to understand any health study." *Vox Science and Health*. January 5, 2015. Accessed August 13 2015. http://www.vox.com/2015/1/5/7482871/types-of-study-design.

[174] Bouchez, Colette. "HRT: Revisiting the Hormone Decision." *WebMD: Menopause Health Center*. Accessed August 13, 2015. http://www.webmd.com/menopause/features/hrt-revisiting-the-hormone-decision.

[175] "Prostate Specific Androgen (PSA) Test." *National Cancer Institute*. July 24, 2012. Accessed August 13, 2015. http://www.cancer.gov/types/prostate/psa-fact-sheet.

[176] Moyer, Melinda W., and Dean Ornish. "Why Almost Everything Dean Ornish Says About Nutrition is Wrong. UPDATED: With Dean Ornish's Response." *Scientific American*, June 1, 2015. Accessed August, 2, 2015. http://www.scientificamerican.com/article/why-almost-everything-dean-ornish-says-about-nutrition-is-wrong/.

[177] "Sleeper." Video, 00:54. *YouTube* Posted October 26 2010. https://www.youtube.com/watch?v=_qto-UwNS-Q.

[178] "*Sleeper*." Directed by Woody Allen. Los Angeles, CA: Rollins-Joffe Productions. 1973.

[179] Perlmutter, David. *Grain Brain*. New York: Little, Brown and Company. 2013.

[180] "Tiger's Milk." *Wikipedia*. September 1 2015. Accessed November 24, 2015. https://en.wikipedia.org/wiki/Tiger%27s_Milk

[181] Forshee, Richard A., Maureen L. Storey, David B. Allison, Walter H. Glinsmann, Gayle L. Hein, David R. Lineback, Sanford A. Miller, et. al. "A critical examination of the evidence relating high fructose corn syrup and weigh gain." *Critical Reviews in Food Science and Nutrition*. 47, no. 6 (2007): 561-582. doi:10.1080/10408390600846457.

[182] Brinkeborn, R. M., D. V. Shah, and F. H. Degenring. "Echinaforce® and other Echinacea fresh plant preparations in the treatment of the common cold: a randomized, placebo controlled, double-blind clinical trial." *Phytomedicine* 6, no. 1 (1999): 1-6. doi:10.1016/S0944-7113(99)80027-0.

[183] Turner, Ronald B., Rudolf Bauer, Karin Woelkart, Thomas C. Hulsey, and J. David Gangemi. "An evaluation of Echinacea angustifolia in experimental rhinovirus infections." *New England Journal of Medicine* 353, no. 4 (2005): 341-348. doi:10.1056/NEJMoa044441.

[184] O'Connor, Anahad. "Coca Cola Funds Scientists Who Shift the Blame for Obesity Away from Bad Diets." *The New York Times: Well* (blog), August 9, 2015. Accessed August 13, 2015. http://well.blogs.nytimes.com/2015/08/09/coca-cola-funds-scientists-who-shift-blame-for-obesity-away-from-bad-diets/?smid=tw-nytimes&_r=0.

[185] Nestle, Marion. "Food Industry Conflicts of Interest: Newspaper Revelations and Five More Studies with Expected Results: The Latest Collection." *Food Politics*. August 10, 2015. Accessed August 13, 2015. http://www.foodpolitics.com/2015/08/food-industry-conflicts-of-interest-newspaper-revelations-and-five-more-studies-with-expected-results-the-latest-collection/.

[186] Janssen, Imke, Alan L. Landay, Kristine Ruppert, and Lynda H. Powell. "Moderate wine consumption is associated with lower hemostatic and inflammatory risk factors over 8 years: The study of women's health across the nation (SWAN)." Nutrition and Aging. 2, no. 2 (2014): 91-99. doi:10.3233/NUA-130034.

In Closing...

[187] Davey, Melissa. "Belle Gibson on 60 Minutes: no remorse and the lies kept coming." *theguardian*. June 28, 2015. Accessed December 19, 2015. http://www.theguardian.com/tv-and-radio/2015/jun/29/belle-gibson-tells-60-minutes-she-was-the-victim-after-her-lies-were-exposed.

Index

Acknowledgements

This book would not be possible without the instruction from and support of many brilliant and talented people.

Dr. John Berardi and his team at Precision Nutrition are the inspiration for the five mantras that make up the Eating component. Without their training, none of this book would be possible.

The instructors at Duke University's Integrative Health Coaching Professional Training Program set me on a course to document a Plan component in which I take particular pride.

Some amazing people had my back and graciously allowed me to pick their brains including my Integrative Health Coach colleagues, Barbara Greco, Sharon Lewis, and Jackie Oken.

Other contributors of content advice and additional support include Alex Ward, Anne Haliday, Arlene Weinstock, Binnie Baumgartner, Cindy and Michael Sauber, David Kim, Tina and George Michallas, Helene Dolan, Ken Friedman, Kirsten Denney, Larry Osman, Marcus Embry, Mike Lau, Nancy Wilborn, Phil Bell, Bob Wright, Robin Barrett, Trip Dubard, Tracy Brennan, and Valerie Rind.

A huge shout out goes to Richard Demler who designed the beautiful cover and Jeanie Simoncic whose editing skills helped turn this hot mess into something readable.

Finally, it may be trite, but I can't thank my partner in crime, Susan enough for her tolerating my foolishness during this process and actually diving in to help when she has her own mega-project(s) to deal with. People who know us know that she stands alone as my reason for wanting to be healthy, always being happy, and oh yeah, putting me in a position to save the world.

The Karma Sense Eating Plan